www.wadsworth.com

wadsworth.com is the World Wide Web site for Wadsworth and is your direct source to dozens of online resources.

At *wadsworth.com* you can find out about supplements, demonstration software, and student resources. You can also send email to many of our authors and preview new publications and exciting new technologies.

wadsworth.com
Changing the way the world learns®

Walking for Fun and Fitness

Third Edition

Jerald D. Hawkins

Lander University

Sandra M. Hawkins

Wellness Consultant

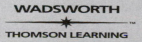

WADSWORTH

TM

THOMSON LEARNING

Australia • Canada • Mexico • Singapore • Spain • United Kingdom • United States

WADSWORTH

THOMSON LEARNING

Publisher: Peter Marshall
Associate Editor: April Lemons
Assistant Editor: John Boyd
Editorial Assistant: Andrea Kesterke
Marketing Manager: Joanne Terhaar
Project Editor: Sandra Craig
Print Buyer: Robert King
Permissions Editor: Stephanie Keough-Hedges
Production and Composition: Ash Street Typecrafters, Inc.
Text and Cover Design: Harry Voigt
Copy Editor: Laura Larson
Printer: Webcom Limited

COPYRIGHT © 2001 Wadsworth, a division of Thomson Learning, Inc.
Thomson Learning™ is a trademark used herein under license.

ALL RIGHTS RESERVED. No part of this work covered by the copyright
hereon may be reproduced or used in any form or by any means—
graphic, electronic, or mechanical, including photocopying, recording,
taping, Web distribution, or information storage and retrieval systems—
without the written permission of the publisher.

ISBN 0-534-58932-4

Printed in Canada
1 2 3 4 5 6 7   04 03 02 01 00

For permission to use material from this text, contact us by
Web: http://www.thomsonrights.com
Fax: 1-800-730-2215
Phone: 1-800-730-2214

Wadsworth/Thomson Learning
10 Davis Drive
Belmont, CA 94002-3098
USA

For more information about our products, contact us:
Thomson Learning Academic Resource Center
1-800-423-0563
http://www.wadsworth.com

International Headquarters
Thomson Learning
International Division
290 Harbor Drive, 2nd Floor
Stamford, CT 06902-7477
USA

UK/Europe/Middle East/South Africa
Thomson Learning
Berkshire House
168-173 High Holborn
London WC1V 7AA
United Kingdom

Asia
Thomson Learning
60 Albert Street, #15-01
Albert Complex
Singapore 189969

Canada
Nelson Thomson Learning
1120 Birchmount Road
Toronto, Ontario M1K 5G4
Canada

Contents

Preface

We believe if you walk for fun and enjoyment, fitness will be your reward. Sound too simple? We know personally, and research supports, that walking has many advantages over other forms of exercise; that is why it is the most popular form of exercise among Americans who exercise regularly. The simple truth is that walking is both fun and a great fitness activity. Throughout this book, we look at many of the reasons why this is so.

- Part One (Chapters 1–3) is an introduction to the nature and benefits of the wonderful activity of walking.

- Part Two (Chapters 4–7) explores the "how to's" of designing and sticking with a fun, effective program. Specific topics include exercise principles, walking mechanics, planning essentials, and motivation and incentive techniques.

- Part Three (Chapters 8–11) deals with issues related to maximizing the effectiveness of your walking program: injury prevention and care, nutrition, weight management, and walking resources.

- The appendices contain personal worksheets for calculating your target heart rate, establishing your walking accountability plan, determining your estimated daily energy expenditure, and charting your walking progress.

As physical educators, former runners and aerobics instructors, and proud and devoted grandparents, we share a commitment to fitness for ourselves and others. Having discovered the myriad of benefits that walking has to offer, this book is our way of sharing both the fun and fitness of walking. Today we are more convinced than ever that if you will avail yourself of the knowledge and use the motivation techniques contained in this book, you, too, will discover that walking truly is *fun*—and if you walk for fun, fitness will come.

Dedication

This book is dedicated to our children,
Lisa, Jennifer, Kiley, and Keri.
We have learned more from them throughout the years
than we have ever taught them.

Thanks, guys—we love you.

Acknowledgments

We express sincere gratitude to Peter Marshall and April Lemons for their guidance and support and to Joanne Saliger for her wonderful creative efforts that truly brought this project to life.

We also give our thanks to a special group of Lander University students who contributed to the success of this book.

About the Authors

Jerald D. Hawkins earned his Ed.D. at the University of Georgia. He is a professor of physical education and exercise studies at Lander University. Recipient of the 1990 South Carolina Association for Health, Physical, Education, Recreation, and Dance College/University Physical Educator of the Year Award, the 1998 Lander University Distinguished Professor award, and the 1999 South Carolina Governor's Professor of the Year award, he is a fellow of the American College of Sports Medicine. Dr. Hawkins is a sought-after speaker and consultant and the author of numerous professional articles, book chapters, and other books.

Sandra M. Hawkins received her M.A.T. from Winthrop University. She is the executive director of the Education Enrichment Foundation of Greenwood County and a former elementary and university physical educator. She served as the first president of the South Carolina Association for Physical Education and Sport and, in 1993, was recognized with that organization's Elementary Physical Educator of the Year Award. She is the author of several articles on fitness walking and creative activities for children.

Together, they provide wellness consultation services, speaking, writing, and conducting workshops on a variety of topics including fitness walking, nutrition, stress management, playground supervision and safety, and legal issues in physical education, exercise, and sport.

Photography by
Joel Nichols, Rock Hill, SC; Bob Stoner, Greenwood, SC;
and the authors

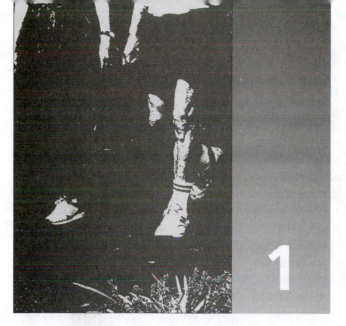

The sum of the whole is this: walk and be happy; walk and be healthy. The best way to lengthen out our days is to walk steadily and with a purpose.
Charles Dickens

1

Introduction

Throughout history, man has used exercise in an attempt to improve athletic performance, prevent illness, recover from injury, slow the aging process, and for a variety of other reasons. While exercise has never been proven to be the cure-all for people's ills that some have touted it to be, exercise-related fitness (often referred to as physical fitness) is universally recognized as an integral part of a healthy lifestyle.

History of Fitness in America

Americans have traditionally had an on again, off again infatuation with exercise and fitness. Sport historians point out that fitness booms tend to follow closely on the heels of our involvement in war. World War I and II and the Korean War all brought with their conclusions a national interest in improved fitness, spurred on by the concern over the physical condition of our troops. Such interest, however, was usually short-lived and tended to wane as the United States returned to the prosperity of peacetime.

During the mid-1960s, America was at war in Southeast Asia, and once again, the fitness of our young people became an issue of major concern. In the wake of this new-found interest, young people and adults alike began engaging in personal exercise programs at a rate never before seen in this country. Jogging, walking, aerobics, and a myriad of other activities became a way of life for millions of Americans. Although initially considered just another fitness fad, it soon became apparent that exercise and exercise-related fitness were concepts whose time had truly come. What may have begun as a fad has become a commitment on the part of millions of Americans to a healthier and more active lifestyle.

In the late 1960s, Dr. Kenneth Cooper, a former Air Force physician, wrote the book *Aerobics* and became the father of the fitness revolution in America. As a result of his extensive research and personal experiences, Cooper has convinced numerous Americans that the key to improved health and fitness is aerobic (cardio-respiratory) exercise. His idea that the quality of our lives in the future will be directly determined by the way we live in the present has been echoed by numerous fitness and medical experts. Simply stated, we have come to understand that living a healthy lifestyle today is an investment in a healthy, enjoyable life in the future.

The 1990s saw the maturing of the baby boomers. Many experts consider this large segment of the U.S. population to be the first generation with a truly conscious commitment to personal health and fitness. Therefore, the motto for many adults in the twenty-first century has become "Fit is in."

What Does "Being Fit" Mean?

The term *fitness* is not easily defined. Many attempts at developing a simple and concise definition have failed. The major problem with defining fitness is that it is not a simple concept. Early attempts at describing fitness were based on the notion that "being fit" means that a person can complete his or her daily routine and still have enough energy to engage in recreational activities. While this may sound reasonable, such a description does little to account for differences in "daily routines." One person's daily routine may be composed primarily of desk work, with very little physical activity, whereas another person may spend most of the day in

relatively strenuous physical activity such as construction work. The construction worker may be less than enthusiastic about rushing to the gym to work out than a friend who works behind the desk, but does this mean he or she is less fit?

From a practical standpoint, fitness is simply the extent to which the body can function efficiently. "Being fit," therefore, means having a healthy body that allows you to enjoy life to its fullest. The concept of health-related fitness may be best understood by looking at the specific components that comprise it: aerobic (or cardiorespiratory) fitness, muscular fitness, and body composition (Figure 1.1).

Aerobic Fitness

Many fitness experts consider aerobic or cardiorespiratory fitness to be the most important single exercise-related health fitness component because of its relationship to the prevention and control of America's number one killer, cardiovascular disease. Every year in the United States, cardiovascular disease (disease of the heart and vascular system) kills almost as many people as all other causes of death combined. What makes this fact even more startling is the realization that many of these cardiovascular deaths could be prevented if only people would make some rather simple, positive lifestyle changes and stick with them. Among those behaviors most directly linked with cardiovascular disease are cigarette smoking, obesity, poor nutrition, and *lack of regular exercise.*

While the precise role of exercise-related fitness in the prevention of cardiovascular disease remains a topic of constant debate, evidence continues to mount that regular aerobic exercise produces positive changes in one's level of aerobic

*1. Aerobic (Cardiorespiratory) Fitness
2. Flexibility
3. Muscular Strength ⎤ **Muscular**
*4. Muscular Endurance ⎦ **Fitness**
*5. Body Composition

* These components are directly affected by regular fitness walking.

Figure 1.1 Components of Health-Related Fitness

fitness that in turn enhance a person's chances of reducing the severity of cardiovascular disease, if not preventing its onset altogether.

Aerobic exercise is exercise that produces positive physiological effects on the heart, blood, vascular system, and lungs. In very simple terms, the body requires energy to carry out its functioning. Energy is necessary for the digestive system to process the food we eat, for the brain to carry on its decision-making processes, and, of course, for the muscles to contract, whether to pick up the morning paper from the yard or lift the feet time after time as we take a pleasant walk around the neighborhood. The body has three ways in which energy can be produced, the most efficient of which is known as *aerobic energy production,* or the utilization of oxygen to produce energy. In a very real sense, the body "prefers" to produce its needed energy aerobically because (1) the energy output from the aerobic system is much more plentiful than that from the two anaerobic systems, and (2) the by-products of aerobic energy production are water and carbon dioxide, both easily metabolized by the body, whereas the major by-product of the main (with respect to exercise) anaerobic energy system is lactic acid, a fatigue-causing

substance. From a health perspective, however, the most important advantage of aerobic fitness is its relationship to the prevention of cardiovascular disease.

Muscular Fitness

Muscular fitness is the second major health fitness component. To be more precise, muscular fitness is really three separate and distinct components that combine to produce a functionally efficient muscular system. All movement produced by the body is the direct result of muscle action. Therefore, we depend on the muscles to provide us with the ability to move as we choose without the fear of injury or undue fatigue. This ability to move efficiently, though often taken for granted, plays a vital role in our daily health and well-being.

Flexibility

The first muscular fitness component is *flexibility,* or the ability of a muscle or muscle group to stretch without injury. With poor flexibility, muscles are susceptible to strains (muscle pulls) ranging in severity from mild pain and aggravation to temporary or extended loss of function requiring bed rest, physician care, and lost work time. Lack of flexibility also has been associated with chronic lower-back pain problems (discussed later). The hamstring muscles (muscle group in the back of the thigh) work with the abdominal muscles to stabilize the pelvic girdle. If flexibility of the hamstrings is not maintained, they will tend to tighten, exaggerating the pelvic tilt allowed by the weak abdominal muscles, further complicating the problem of chronic lower-back pain.

The old adage "Use it or lose it" is never more appropriate than when referring to flexibility. Children are generally very flexible, as noted when an infant chews on his toe or puts her foot behind her head. This flexibility, however, is usually short-lived unless the child remains active and engages in flexibility-related activities such as gymnastics or wrestling. As adults, we can lose flexibility rather rapidly unless we make a conscious effort to maintain it. In short, flexibility does not have to dissipate with age, but it often does because of a simple lack of exercise.

Muscular Strength

The second component of muscular fitness is muscular strength. Muscular strength is simply the ability of a muscle or muscle group to contract forcefully against a resistance. Strength is generally more directly associated with athletic prowess than with health fitness, though it is widely accepted that everyone needs a modicum of muscular strength to function effectively on a day-to-day basis, especially if the daily routine requires lifting, pushing, pulling, or carrying heavy objects.

There is an even more direct link between muscular strength and health fitness for the general population. The abdominal muscles act to stabilize the pelvic girdle. When they are fit and strong, the pelvic girdle is maintained in its natural position. However, when the abdominal muscles become weak and out of shape, the pelvic girdle is allowed to tilt abnormally, placing stress on the lower back. This condition may, over time, lead to chronic lower-back pain, a problem all too common today. Often, such pain may be reduced or even eliminated through regular abdominal strengthening exercises, such as bent-knee abdominal curls (sit-ups). Probably the most common type of muscular strength exercise is weight training—the systematic lifting of free weights or work with other devices designed to produce muscular strength gains.

Muscular Endurance

Muscular endurance, the ability of a muscle or muscle group to contract repeatedly without undue fatigue, is the final muscular fitness component. To illustrate, one of the first problems encountered by a person when he or she initiates a walking or jogging program is how rapidly the legs become fatigued. This is because the muscles are not accustomed to the stress of repetitive work and are easily tired. Like strength, endurance is often associated more with athletic performance (e.g., distance running) than with health fitness. Muscular fatigue, however, can make even a leisurely walk in the mall an unpleasant experience.

Unlike strength, endurance is most effectively developed through systematically engaging in exercise requiring the muscles to work repetitively against moderate resistance. Such activities as walking, jogging, and bicycling are excellent for improving muscular endurance (as well as circulation) in the legs.

Body Composition

The final major component of exercise-related health fitness is body composition, which is simply a person's relative amount of fat versus fat-free weight. The human body is composed of many types of tissue—muscle, bone, blood, and fat, just to name a few. To function efficiently, the body needs a requisite amount of fat, since fat plays a vital role in the conduction of nerve impulses, insulation and protection of vital organs, utilization of fat-soluble vitamins, and maintenance of healthy skin. This fat is referred to as *essential fat.* The body generally stores additional fat to be used for energy should the need arise. This fat is often referred to as *expendable fat.* When one's fat stores become excessive, the results are health-threatening and may include the inability to regulate body temperature normally; the tendency toward diabetes; stress on the lower back, knees, and ankles, leading to chronic orthopedic problems; and stress on the cardiorespiratory system, resulting in an enhanced probability of cardiovascular disease. In fact, the medical community now considers obesity a disease in itself. (For a more detailed discussion of body composition and weight management, see Chapter 10.)

The surest path to personal fitness and wellness is a commitment to a healthy lifestyle, one characterized by eating right, not smoking or abusing drugs, managing stress, and exercising on a regular basis. What more enjoyable way to exercise our way to fitness than walking?

Walking: A Brief History

Since the dawn of creation, humans have used walking as a practical and inexpensive means of transportation. It has been suggested that walking has been a popular activity ever since people first had somewhere to go and a need for some way to get there. Most Americans can remember when children walked to school, many adults walked to work, and a stroll around the block was a regular after-dinner event.

However, transportation is only one of many ways in which walking has become an integral part of our world. Walking contests were popular in Europe for hundreds of years before being introduced in the United States in the 1870s. They became commonplace in America, with early races often featuring six-day marathon events on indoor oval walking tracks. Race walkers were among the most celebrated athletes of the time. In 1909, Edward Payson Weston walked from San Francisco to New York City in 104 days. Today, many walking enthusiasts consider Rob Sweetgall America's premier fitness walker, having walked 11,600 miles in 363 days in what he called his "50-State Walk for the Health of It."

The most recent survey of fitness and leisure activities by the National Sporting Goods Association, one of the nation's leading sources of market research, indicates that walking is the most popular aerobic fitness activity in the United States today. Among the survey's list of most popular sport and fitness activities, walking ranked number one with nearly 81 million participants (Figure 1.2). People are discovering that walking is both fun and effective for improving fitness through aerobic development, muscular

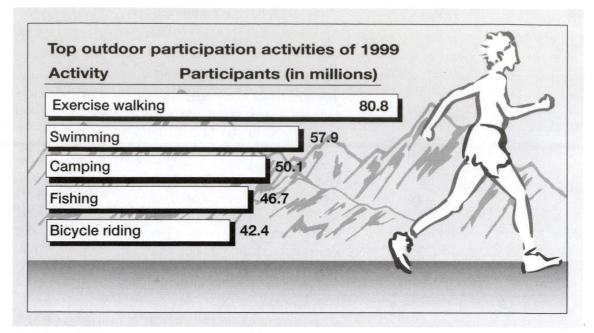

Figure 1.2 Walking: America's Most Popular Fitness Activity

improvement, stress management, and weight control. What's more, the risk of injury is significantly less with walking than with most other forms of exercise. These and other factors have elevated walking to "most popular fitness activity" status in America.

Types of Walking

Not all people who walk do so for their health. Many simply walk for the fun of it, for the sheer enjoyment of getting outdoors into the fresh air. While all walking is beneficial, the pace and regularity of one's walking will determine the extent to which desirable fitness improvements are likely to occur. Therefore, it may be helpful to take a look at the various types of walking one may choose to do (Figure 1.3).

Strolling

Strolling is the term most often used to describe casual walking. Generally done at an easy pace of slower than 3 miles per hour (20 minutes per mile), strolling is great for a person who is recovering from illness or who wishes to begin a walking program after having been sedentary for quite some time. Regardless of the purpose, strolling is most effective when it is done at a pace that will allow walking non-stop for 30 minutes or longer.

For those in reasonably good physical condition, strolling will do little to enhance aerobic fitness. Therefore, one of the following types of "walking with a purpose" should be used. The specific type of walking chosen will depend on the walker's physical condition and the purpose for which the walking is done.

Type	Pace
Strolling	Less than 3 mph (20:00 min/mile)
Fitness walking	3–6 mph (12:00–20:00 min/mile)
Power walking	3–6 mph (12:00–20:00 min/mile) with exaggerated arm swing, hand weights or other external resistance, or both
Race walking	7.5 mph (8:00 min/mile) or faster using prescribed race walking technique

Figure 1.3 Types of Walking

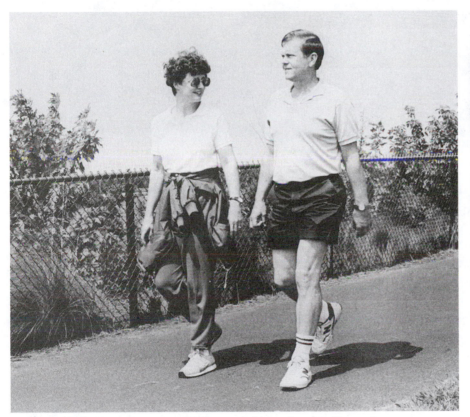

Strolling is casual walking, generally at a pace slower than 3 miles per hour.

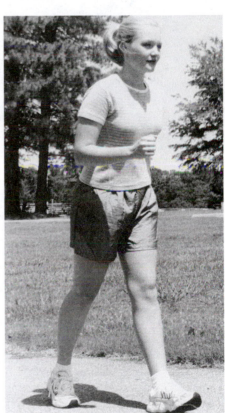

Fitness walking involves a more purposeful stride and arm swing.

Fitness Walking

Fitness walking is the type of walking commonly done to improve one's aerobic fitness level. It is characterized by a longer, faster, more purposeful stride and arm swing than strolling, at a pace of 3 to 6 miles per hour (10 to 20 minutes per mile). This pace is generally sufficient to elevate the heart rate to the desirable aerobic conditioning level and maintain it there throughout the walk.

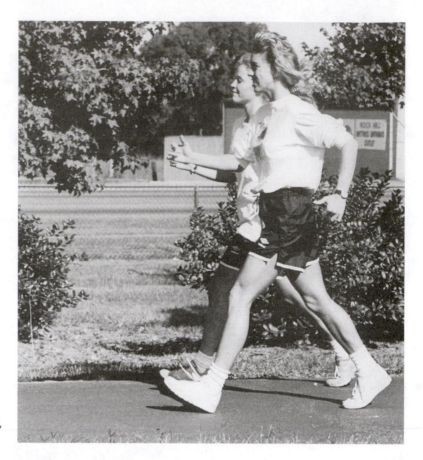

Power walking uses an exaggerated arm swing, hand weights, or both.

Power Walking

Power walking has been compared to cross-country skiing without the skis. While done at the same pace as fitness walking (3 to 6 miles per hour), power walking enthusiasts intensify the effects of the exercise by using exaggerated arm swing and hand weights or other external props, or both.

Race Walking

Despite its somewhat odd appearance, race walking is basically just an accelerated form of normal walking in which speed is the main goal. Race walkers are primarily competitive athletes whose technique must comply with specific rules of the sport. Race walking is typically done at a pace of 7.5 to 9 miles per hour (6.5 to 8 minutes per mile). A detailed discussion of various walking techniques is presented in Chapter 5.

Summary

More health-conscious today than in years past, Americans are exercising in greater numbers than ever before. Health-related fitness is a combination of aerobic (cardiorespiratory) fitness, muscular fitness (flexibility, strength, and endurance), and body composition.

Because of the serious threat that cardiovascular disease continues to pose, aerobic fitness may be called the most important single health-related fitness component.

Therefore, it is important that you engage in regular aerobic exercise, and fitness walking (3 to 6 miles per hour) is one of the most popular and enjoyable of all aerobic activities.

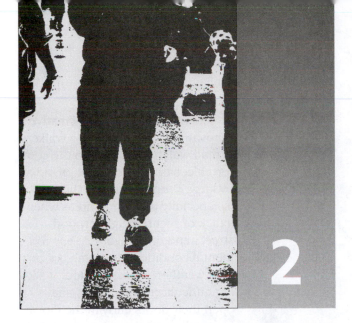

Of all exercise, walking is the best.
Thomas Jefferson

2

Walking: Nature's Most Perfect Exercise?

Throughout the history of sport, fitness, and play, people have searched for "the perfect exercise"—that single activity that will provide maximum health benefits in a wide variety of specific areas while, at the same time, being convenient, inexpensive, safe, painless, and, above all, fun.

Today, Americans are jogging, swimming, skiing, bicycling, dancing, and, yes, walking their way to better health. All of these popular activities are excellent choices for improving aerobic fitness. Each one, when done for 20 to 30 minutes or longer within one's target heart rate range (see Chapter 4), three to five times per week, will lead to an improvement in aerobic fitness. However, if there is one single form of aerobic exercise that deserves the title "nature's most perfect exercise," it just may be walking. For, while many activities can be both fun and effective for improving one's fitness, few

can rival walking for its appeal to people of all ages, convenience, expense, safety, and enjoyment.

Practical Advantages of Walking

Walking Can Be Enjoyed by People of All Ages

Few exercise activities are appropriate for children, young adults, and senior citizens alike. Unlike jogging, running, bicycling, and sports activities like basketball and tennis, walking does not require specialized skills that are not easily mastered by young children. Therefore, a child can begin enjoying the many benefits of walking at an early age—literally, when he or she learns to walk. On the other end of the spectrum, because of its high degree of safety and universal enjoyment, walking is the most popular fitness activity

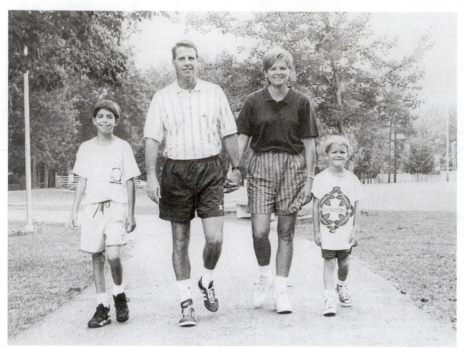

Walking can be enjoyed by people of all ages.

streets and sidewalks of familiar neighborhoods.

One of the more recent creative innovations of some fitness walkers is mall walking, walking in the comfortable, safe environment provided by large shopping malls. This option is especially popular in areas where a lack of secure neighborhood streets and/or unfavorable environmental conditions (extreme hot or cold weather) makes outdoor walking difficult. In some cities, malls open their doors early in the morning to allow walkers use of the mall prior to the opening of the stores, and some even support the formation of mall walking clubs. For the employee who finds lunch hour the best time to walk, sidewalks, parking lots, and even long corridors may be used.

among senior citizens. It is safe to say that walking is probably the only type of exercise that may be enjoyed from ages 2 to 102.

Walking Can Be Done Virtually Anytime, Anywhere

Walking is surely the most convenient of all exercise forms, since it can be done with little or no special considerations of time or location. For some, a brisk walk in the cool of early morning is the perfect way to start a day, while for others, the peace and solitude of an evening walk provides much-needed relief from the rigors of a busy day. For many whose mornings and evenings are filled with other activities, the lunch hour and/or other break times during the day provide excellent walking opportunities. Also, walking can be enjoyed in almost any location. The morning and evening walkers may get special enjoyment from walking in a scenic public park or may simply prefer to walk the

Walking Is Inexpensive

One of the most common reasons cited by people who do not exercise regularly is the cost of exercise equipment, clothing, and spa or club membership fees. With the exception of a good, comfortable pair of shoes, walking requires very little monetary investment. To paraphrase a familiar sales pitch, walking is an activity that can be enjoyed for only pennies a day.

Walking Is Less Likely to Result in Injury Than Most Other Forms of Exercise

One of the most appealing aspects of fitness walking is that it is virtually injury-free. Because one foot is always in contact with the walking surface, less stress is placed on the weight-supporting structures of the feet, ankles, knees, hips, and lower back. While it is undoubtedly true that higher-intensity activities such as running and aerobic dance may yield fitness benefits at a faster rate

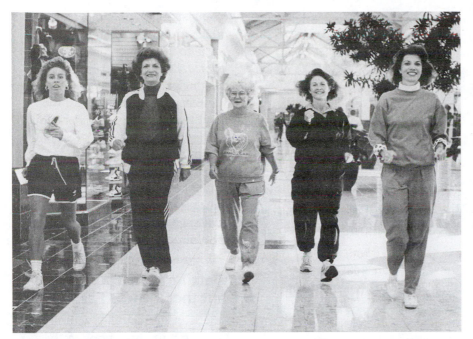

Mall walking has become a popular activity.

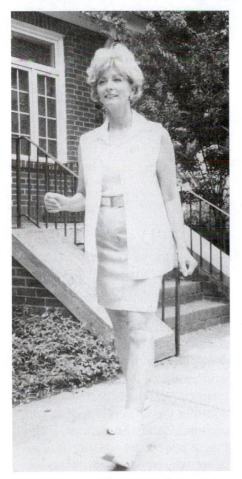

Other than a good pair of shoes, no special equipment is needed for walking.

Walking Is Fun

It is commonly estimated that fewer than 4 of every 10 adult Americans exercise regularly. A wide variety of reasons explain why most Americans choose not to exercise, not the least of which is that many believe that *exercise* and *fun* are mutually exclusive words; in other words, they are convinced that exercise simply cannot be enjoyable. One of the most exciting facts about fitness walking is that it *is* fun.

Whether done at a leisurely pace to simply unwind from a busy day or "walking with a purpose" to develop aerobic fitness and/or control weight, in the stillness of the early morning or the cool of the evening, with a group of friends or alone, walking can be fun.

than walking, these activities are also much more likely to result in injuries that may cause a person to give up exercising altogether. (Specific suggestions for preventing and managing exercise-related injuries are presented in Chapter 8.)

Walking Is Painless

Despite what many people believe, exercise does not need to be painful to be beneficial. For too long, fitness enthusiasts have rallied around the cry "No pain, no gain." While the basic idea that exercise benefits are not realized without physical effort is accurate, the implication that physical effort must be painful has discouraged many a potential exerciser from enjoying the many benefits that regular exercise has to offer. When the body hurts, it is simply sending a message to slow down, and, if these messages are ignored, injury may result. Therefore, the fitness walker would do well to adopt a more sensible motto—"Train, don't strain."

Walking Is a Great Fitness Activity

In addition to being a safe, inexpensive, and enjoyable form of exercise, walking is simply a great way to develop and maintain overall fitness. A regular walking program that includes appropriate warm-up and cool-down activities can positively influence four of the five major components of health-related fitness identified in Chapter 1— aerobic fitness, flexibility, muscular endurance, and body composition. Few fitness activities can make that claim.

Myths and Misconceptions About Walking

Few of us can remember a time in our lives when we did not know how to walk. Consequently, like eating and breathing, walking is something most people take for granted. It should not be surprising, therefore, that some may view the very suggestion of walking as a fitness activity with a great deal of skepticism. As with most issues concerning fitness, the facts about walking as a beneficial and enjoyable fitness activity are often distorted by myths and misconceptions. The following are some of the most common erroneous beliefs of walking critics.

Walking Isn't Real Exercise; It's Just Walking

Those who see walking as something less than "real exercise" may simply observe that "Everyone walks, everyday; so why isn't everyone fit?" As stated in Chapter 1, the answer to this rather logical-sounding question is that not all walking is fitness walking. However, fitness walking is real exercise that produces real fitness benefits—and lots of them, including improved aerobic fitness, enhanced muscular endurance, weight control, and effective stress management. (Specific effects of fitness walking are discussed in Chapter 3.) However, most fitness experts agree with the noted surgeon and sports medicine specialist, Dr. Saul Haskell, who observed, "Anything you can accomplish running, you can accomplish walking. It just takes a little longer."

Walking Is Boring

Who says? Yes, even the most perfect exercise can be boring, if the participant lacks the creativity to keep the fun and challenge alive. And yes, fitness walking, like any type of exercise, can become monotonous in spite of all its great physical and psychological benefits. However, it has been said that people who are easily bored are usually boring people. While this may be a somewhat unfair generalization, it does imply that boredom,

in any situation, is largely a matter of personal choice. Therefore, the key is to look for creative ways to keep walking an interesting, even exciting part of your lifestyle. For some people, knowledge of the many benefits of walking is enough to keep them on a regular walking program, while others practice a wide variety of self-motivation techniques to add enjoyment to their routine (see Chapter 7). The challenge is to create your walking program just the way you want it.

Walking Is Just Another Fitness Fad

Americans are familiar with fitness fads, from the hula hoop to the pogo stick. A *fad* is a product or idea that enjoys immense popularity for a short time and then quickly loses its appeal when the novelty wears off. Fitness walking is the exercise of choice of one out of four Americans who exercise. With more than 80 million Americans regularly participating in fitness walking, it is fair to say that walking is not just another fitness fad but a fitness activity that has found its place in the hearts, minds, and "soles" of the American public.

Summary

No single form of exercise can develop total fitness. However, a regular walking program can have a positive impact on aerobic fitness, muscular endurance, and body composition. When warm-up and cool-down stretching is added to your program, flexibility improvement can also be expected. If you consider the universal appeal, convenience, safety, enjoyment, and fitness benefits of walking, it is easy to see why walking may just be "nature's most perfect exercise."

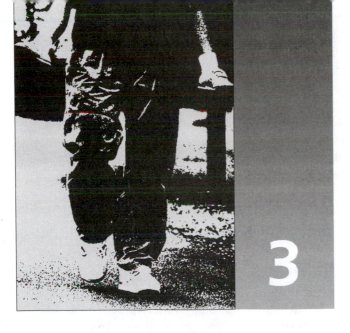

It is solved by walking.

Latin proverb

3

Why Walking?

To suggest that every problem can be solved simply by walking may be a bit of an overstatement. However, it is true that the advantages offered by fitness walking are virtually endless. In this chapter we will take a closer look at some of the specific benefits you can enjoy as a fitness walker.

Improved Aerobic Fitness

Walking is an excellent aerobic activity. Simply stated, regular fitness walking can produce a variety of positive changes in your cardiovascular and respiratory systems.

Stronger, More Elastic Heart Muscle

The heart is basically a hollow muscle that serves as a pump to circulate blood. Regular aerobic exercise such as walking causes the heart muscle to become both stronger and more elastic. The result of these changes is an increase in the amount of blood that your heart can pump, since a stronger heart can contract more forcefully and a more elastic heart muscle can expand to accept more blood when it fills.

Increased Stroke Volume

Each time the heart contracts (beats), it pumps oxygen-rich blood out to the body tissues. The amount of blood pumped with each beat is known as the heart's *"stroke volume."* The increased strength and elasticity of the heart muscle produced by aerobic exercise enables the heart to pump more blood with each beat.

Decreased Resting Heart Rate

Heart rate (often called *pulse*) is the number of times your heart beats each minute. As you become more aerobically fit, your resting heart rate will tend to decrease, since the stronger and more elastic heart can pump more blood with each contraction (beat), thus requiring fewer contractions (beats) to meet the body's demand for oxygen-rich blood.

Increased Heart Efficiency

In the same way that your automobile requires fuel (gasoline) to run, your heart requires fuel (oxygen) to pump the blood your body needs. As aerobic fitness improves, the heart is able to pump more blood while requiring less oxygen to pump that blood. One major reason for this is that the heart requires less energy to contract more forcefully, fewer times than to contract less forcefully but faster. Therefore, the increased stroke volume and decreased heart rate discussed earlier produce a more efficiently functioning heart.

Stronger, More Elastic Blood Vessels

The body contains three major types of blood vessels: arteries (which carry blood away from the heart), veins (which return blood to the heart), and capillaries (which allow the exchange of oxygen and carbon dioxide between blood and tissues). One of the major positive changes produced by aerobic exercise is that these vascular structures become stronger and more elastic. As a result, the vessels are more resistant to the constant pressure of blood flowing through them.

Increased Active Capillary Density

Each of us has millions of capillaries in our body, but most (possibly as many as 95%) are inactive. Regular aerobic exercise such as walking produces a systematic increase in the number of active capillaries, especially in those muscle groups used in the activity. As the number of active capillaries increases, so does the capacity for oxygen delivery to that area.

Decreased Blood Pressure

Arteries are under constant pressure from the blood being circulated through them. Improved vascular elasticity, coupled with increased numbers of active capillaries, lessens blood pressure both at rest and during exercise. This allows the arteries to accommodate more blood with less pressure-induced stress. Lowered resting blood pressure is a common indicator of aerobic fitness.

Improved Capillary Diffusion

One of the determining factors for efficient oxygen and carbon dioxide exchange is the extent to which capillaries allow gas diffusion to occur. With improved aerobic fitness, capillaries become more receptive to the diffusion of oxygen and carbon dioxide, making the exchange of these gases in the lungs and muscles more efficient.

Improved Venous Return

When blood is pumped out to the muscles through the arteries, it must return to the heart through the venous (veins) system. From the extremities (especially the legs), blood must overcome gravity to make its way back to the heart. One way in which the body assists the blood in its return to the heart is through the "milking" action of contracting muscles. As you walk, the major muscles of the legs rhythmically contract and relax, creating a pumping action on the veins they surround. As a result, blood is forced upward toward the heart. As you become more fit, the muscles will develop an improved "tone" that will provide support for the veins and improved blood return even at rest.

Improved Coronary Blood Flow

As mentioned earlier, the heart muscle must have oxygen to function. This oxygen is provided through blood circulated to the heart muscle by the coronary (heart) arteries. Regular aerobic exercise improves blood flow to the heart muscle by increasing the size and efficiency of the coronary vessels and possibly by resulting in the formation of small coronary artery branches, though research in this area is inconclusive.

Increased Blood Volume

In addition to the beneficial effects on the heart and blood vessels, walking can also improve both the quantity and quality of your blood. Regular aerobic exercise has been shown to increase the amount of blood in the body. This enables you to maintain a desirable heart-filling pressure during exercise.

Improved Blood Lipid Profile

Your blood contains a variety of lipids (fats and fatlike substances), including triglycerides (fats) and cholesterol. Excessive amounts of blood triglycerides and certain types of cholesterol have been linked to cardiovascular disease. Regular aerobic exercise can alter your blood lipid profile in several positive ways. First, the amount of circulating triglycerides (fats) may decrease. Second, you may lower the total amount of blood cholesterol.

Third, and possibly most important, the amount of HDL (high-density lipoprotein) cholesterol in the blood increases with regular aerobic exercise. HDL cholesterol has been called "good cholesterol" because of its apparent protective role in the development of coronary artery disease. Although the exact mechanism is unclear, it is clear that raising the HDL cholesterol level in the blood can provide some protection against cardiovascular disease, and regular aerobic exercise has been shown to increase HDL levels.

Increased Lung Function

Under normal circumstances, the body can take in enough air to provide the oxygen it needs. However, walking and other forms of aerobic exercise enable the lungs to fill and empty more fully, thus increasing the amount of air the lungs can exchange and improving the ease and efficiency with which this exchange takes place.

Increased Aerobic Capacity

The best overall indicator of aerobic fitness is *"aerobic capacity,"* the maximum ability of the body to take in, transport, absorb, and utilize oxygen for energy. As you become more aerobically fit, you will find it easier to walk for longer distances and at a faster pace, because the body will gradually increase its ability to work aerobically under more demanding conditions. This is simply the collective, "bottom line" effect of the specific individual changes discussed earlier. Although increased aerobic capacity can be accurately measured through sophisticated lab testing, you need look no further than the greater ease and enjoyment of your daily walk to appreciate the aerobic benefits of walking.

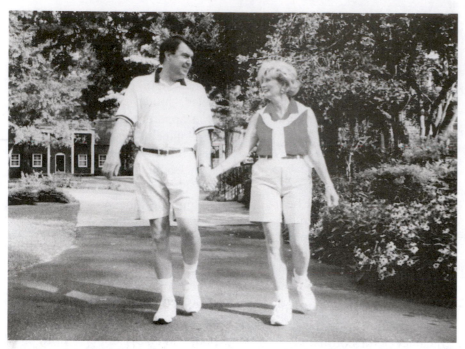

Walking is a great way to share quality time with family and friends.

increase in active capillary density discussed previously and an improvement in the aerobic metabolism of individual muscle fibers (cells). Simply stated, the muscle fibers adapt to the demands of regular exercise.

Increased Energy

As you become more aerobically fit, your body will require less energy to function efficiently. Therefore, you will find that you have more energy and vigor for both work and play. Aside from the other numerous physical benefits of a walking program, many people simply cite more energy and feeling better as their main reasons for walking.

Improved Muscular Endurance

As discussed in Chapter 1, muscular endurance is the ability of a muscle or muscle group to contract repeatedly without fatigue. As you begin your walking program, you may notice that your legs tire easily. This is because the muscles are unaccustomed to repetitive work. As you increase the regularity of your walking, you will notice that the muscles will become more energetic and resistant to fatigue. Although a host of factors contribute to this change, the most prominent involve the

Improved Flexibility

Walking itself will do little to improve the flexibility (elasticity) of the muscles. In fact, as you walk, the weight-supporting muscles of the legs will actually tend to tighten. However, the use of stretching exercises (like those recommended in Chapter 7) before and after your walk will increase the elasticity of the individual muscle fibers and connective tissue, resulting in a desirable improvement in flexibility.

Increased Bone Density

Even the bones benefit from a regular walking program. Walking (and other weight-bearing exercise) has been shown to increase the density and strength of bones. It is believed that regular exercise may be an important factor in preventing or lessening the effects of such disabling bone disorders as osteoporosis.

Improved Immune Function

One of the most important assets of the human body is its ability to resist disease. Through a complex process known collectively as the body's immune system, your body routinely fights off disease-causing organisms. With the recent emergence of AIDS and other immune deficiency conditions, we have all become aware of the importance of a strong immune system. Recent research indicates that regular aerobic

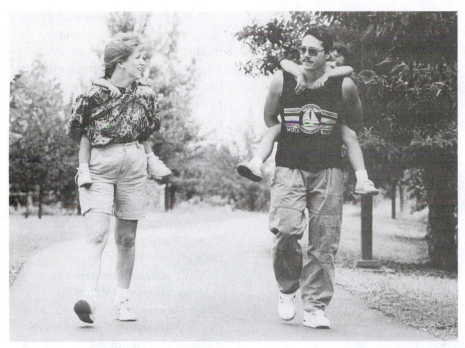

Walking is an excellent family activity.

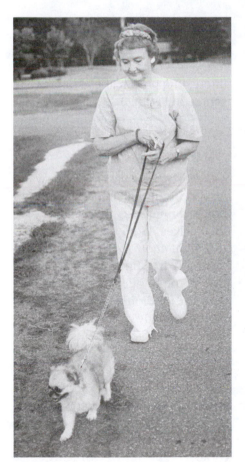

Even walking your dog can become a fun fitness activity.

accomplishment, and walking is an exercise that makes "sticking with it" easy. In only a short time, you will begin to experience the positive effects of exercise, and you will begin to feel better. When the benefits begin to show up in the form of a healthier body, you can't help but feel better about yourself.

Weight Control

Regular aerobic exercise is a vital factor in maintaining a desirable body weight, and walking specifically is an enjoyable and effective weight control exercise. A detailed discussion of weight management is presented in Chapter 10.

exercise strengthens the body's immune system, which, in turn, means fewer and less severe infectious diseases.

Reduced Stress

Many people find walking a great way to reduce stress. The opportunity to get outside and release pent-up tension is a wonderful way to cope with the stresses of daily life. Walking can provide some quiet, relaxed thinking time—often a missing ingredient in our busy schedule. Aerobic exercise may also help alleviate stress by producing a positive change in brain chemistry. This is why aerobic exercise has often been called a "natural high."

Improved Self-Esteem

It is not difficult to see how self-esteem can be enhanced by participating in a regular exercise program. Making and keeping a commitment to exercise regularly can provide a real sense of

Improved Appearance

Regular walking can simply result in a better-looking you. In addition to its role in weight loss and maintenance, walking has also been shown to improve overall muscle tone, improve skin appearance by improving superficial circulation, and foster better posture. These results not only are positive health effects but will contribute to a better overall appearance. Also, when you feel good, you project a more positive image.

Fun

In addition to walking's many health and fitness benefits, it is simply fun. Doing something that is good for you provides a sense of accomplishment, and, for some, this is the real fun of walking. For others, walking where they can greet and talk with friends or neighbors or simply have an opportunity to enjoy the beauty of nature makes walking more than just good exercise.

Consider these reasons—some serious, some humorous, but all true.

1. Have fun.
2. Improve your aerobic fitness.
3. Increase your energy.
4. Improve your muscular endurance.
5. Improve your flexibility.
6. Increase your bone density.
7. Reduce tension and manage stress.
8. Enjoy a sense of accomplishment.
9. Lose/maintain weight.
10. Look better and feel better.
11. Enjoy quality time with your family/friends.
12. Meet new friends and neighbors.
13. Fight the desire to smoke.
14. Enjoy the beauties of nature.
15. Walk your dog (or your friend's dog).
16. Bird watch, people watch, or both.
17. Engage in some creative thinking.
18. Impress your friends and neighbors.
19. Be a fitness role model.
20. Enjoy your favorite music.
21. Memorize class notes, Bible verses, etc.
22. Get away from the telephone (only works if you don't carry one with you).

Your favorites? _____

_____

_____

Figure 3.1 Why Walk?

For many people, walking provides an opportunity to share quality time with a friend or family member without the interruption of the telephone, television, or other modern "conveniences." Walking is also a great time to listen to favorite music in the serenity of nature. Small children often enjoy the many special sights, sounds, and smells that can be found during a walk. Like many walkers, you may simply find the pleasure of peaceful thought and relaxation enjoyment enough.

Give yourself the freedom to create your own walking fun. Suggestions for helping you create fun in your walking program are presented in Chapter 7.

Other Benefits

Regular fitness walking offers numerous other benefits. Some interesting possibilities are presented in Figure 3.1.

Summary

The reasons people choose to walk and continue walking are as numerous and unique as the walkers themselves. From improved fitness, to weight control, stress reduction, or simply fun, fitness walking has something to offer virtually everyone. The cardiorespiratory, muscular, body composition, and psychological benefits of regular aerobic exercise are well documented. Therefore, if you are interested in exercising your way to looking better, feeling better, and simply living a fuller, more enjoyable life, fitness walking is an excellent choice.

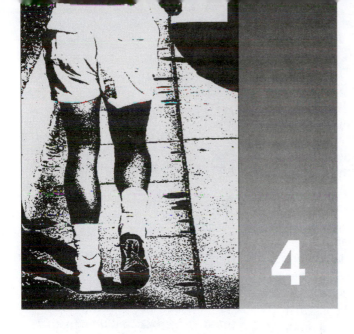

4

Take a two-mile walk every morning before breakfast.

Harry S. Truman

Exercise Principles and Fitness Walking

A successful walking program depends, to a great extent, on understanding and applying a few basic principles. A *principle* is simply a guideline or recommendation that, if followed, improves your chances of enjoying success. Just as the building of a house is guided by certain principles of design and construction, an effective walking program must be based on sound principles of exercise. Although the following exercise principles are set forth in rather specific terms, you should never lose sight of the fact that they must be used within the bounds of common sense—more of a good thing is not always better or even advisable.

SAID Principle

The SAID (specific adaptation to imposed demands) principle states that the body will respond directly to those physical demands placed on it by adapting to those demands in a rather predictable manner. When aerobic demands are placed on the body, the cardiorespiratory system will adapt to those demands by becoming stronger and more efficient. Conversely, if aerobic demands are not systematically placed on the cardiorespiratory system, the body's adaptation will be in the form of lost conditioning. Therefore, walking, because of its aerobic nature, can be expected to result in an improvement in cardiorespiratory fitness if done according to the principles of prescription presented in this chapter.

Principle of Overload

The overload principle states that for improvement to occur in any physiological system, that system must be placed under training demands that are greater than the normal demands encountered by that system on a daily basis. For example, a program for muscular strength development must systematically require the muscles to work against a resistance level that is greater than that with which they are routinely faced. Similarly, you must progressively walk at a faster pace and/or for a longer period of time (or distance) than normally experienced in your daily routine, since systematic increases in exercise time and/or pace are necessary to challenge the cardiovascular system appropriately and produce the desired results.

Principle of Progression

The principle of progression could easily be called the "principle of common sense," because it describes the body's need to face increased physical demands in a gradual and systematic manner. When initiating a walking program, you should begin at a comfortable pace and walk for a comfortable period of time or distance. As the body becomes accustomed to the exercise, the pace and/or duration of the walk should be gradually increased.

Principle of Specificity

The principle of specificity states that the results of an exercise program will directly reflect the type of exercise done. While weight training is an effective way to improve muscular strength, it does little to improve aerobic fitness. Therefore, an aerobic activity such as walking must be used if cardiorespiratory fitness is the expected outcome. Simply stated, an exercise will do only those things that it is designed to do.

Principle of Detraining

The principle of detraining describes how the body responds to inactivity. Just as the body's cardiovascular and respiratory systems will become stronger and more efficient through systematic training, the heart, vascular system, blood, lungs, and other related structures will begin to deteriorate when you cease exercising. It would be nice if a certain level of fitness could be attained through exercise and then maintained throughout life without further effort. However, the shocking fact is that the decline in fitness that accompanies inactivity usually occurs at a much more rapid rate than did the exercise-induced gains—often twice as rapidly. Therefore, an exercise program must be maintained if the benefits gained from the program are to be maintained—"use it or lose it."

Principle of Overtraining

The principle of overtraining recognizes the fact that too much of a good thing can be detrimental. As discussed later in this chapter, the body will respond most favorably to exercise when it is done in the recommended manner, but it will respond negatively if training is done too intensely, too long, too fast, or too often. The effects of overtraining can include chronic fatigue, difficulty sleeping, poor appetite, or even needless injury or illness. Fortunately, however, because of the low impact and moderate intensity associated with walking, the danger of experiencing overtraining is less likely with fitness walking than with most other types of fitness exercise.

Principle of Individual Differences

The principle of individual differences states that no two people will respond to a particular type of exercise program in exactly the same manner. Although fitness walking will produce specific aerobic physiological adaptations in the cardiovascular system, how much improvement you can expect is at least partially determined by your innate physical capacity. Failure to recognize that everyone does not progress at the same rate may lead to needless frustration for a person who exercises long and hard but does not improve as rapidly as a friend who follows the same exercise regimen. For this reason, each person must walk at the pace and progress at the rate that is best suited to his or her individual needs and abilities. You should not compare your fitness status, therefore, to that of friends whose programs are designed to meet their own unique needs.

Principles of Prescription

If your physician gave you a medication with the instructions "Take as many of these as you need to cure the illness, but not too many, or too often, or for too long," what would you do? Obviously, such haphazard instructions would produce confusion, at the very least, and possibly hazardous results. To be effective and safe, exercise, like medication, should be carefully prescribed and "taken" according to the recommended prescription. Four principles state that the effectiveness and safety of a specific exercise program will be directly related to

1. the type of exercise done (principle of mode or type),
2. how hard the individual exercises (principle of intensity),
3. how long the individual exercises (principle of duration), and
4. how often the individual exercises (principle of frequency).

As stated in Chapter 2, walking, along with the stretching exercises done during warm-up and cool-down, will have a positive effect on not only aerobic efficiency but flexibility, muscular endurance, and body composition as well. Therefore, the four principles of prescription must be understood as they apply to each of these major fitness components.

Type (What Type of Exercise Should I Do?)

As discussed earlier, the specific type(s) of exercise chosen will depend directly on the desired results of the exercise program. For the improvement or maintenance of aerobic efficiency, the exercise program should be built around an aerobic activity such as walking.

Improved flexibility can be best accomplished through static stretching. The specific stretching activities chosen will depend on the specific muscle groups in which flexibility improvement is desired. A good rule of thumb, however, is that flexibility improvement should involve all major muscle groups, with special emphasis placed on those muscle groups used most frequently in daily work, recreational, and fitness activities. Some recommended stretching activities are presented in Chapter 7.

Muscular endurance is improved by contracting a muscle or muscle group repeatedly against a moderate resistance. This is why walking is such a good way to develop muscular endurance in the legs. While walking, the major muscle groups in the legs contract and relax rhythmically with every stride, while supporting your body weight.

As will be discussed in Chapter 10, weight (body composition) management requires a combination of dietary modification and exercise. For this purpose, aerobic activities like walking have been shown to be the most effective, because of their ability to provide efficient caloric expenditure over an extended period of time.

The selection of specific activities should also be based on such personal considerations as interest and convenience. Since you are more likely to take part in an activity that you find personally interesting, it makes sense to select activities that offer the greatest amount of personal interest and enjoyment. With this in mind, walking would appear an ideal choice.

Convenience is also a factor that must be considered if the selected activity is to become a part of your lifestyle. Having to drive 10 minutes to a swimming pool after a hard day at the office may soon become more trouble than it is worth, while the same benefits may be gained by walking to a neighborhood park for a long, scenic walk.

Intensity (How Hard Should I Exercise?)

One of the greatest disservices done to the would-be exerciser by so-called "fitness experts" is the promotion of the catchy phrase "No pain, no gain!" As noted earlier, exercise does not have to be painful to be effective. In fact, many a sincere desire to exercise has been squelched by frustration and injury resulting from the unfortunate, and often dangerous, misconception that exercise must hurt to be beneficial. While it is true that exercise generally does produce elevated body temperature, perspiration, fatigue, and occasionally muscle soreness, fitness-related exercise should be an enjoyable experience, not a painful one.

The recommended intensity for aerobic exercise can be very simply calculated and personalized using your resting and exercise heart rates (pulse) as an indicator. You can monitor your heart rate easily by placing two fingers on the Adam's apple and sliding them into the natural groove on the side of the neck (carotid pulse). Then count your pulse for 10 seconds and multiply that number by 6. One recommended method for determining your appropriate aerobic exercise intensity is presented in Figures 4.1 and 4.2 and Appendix A.

These individuals' heart rates (144 to 158 for the example male and 152 to 164 for the example female) are the target heart rate ranges (THRRs) within which their walking should be done for maximum aerobic benefit. Once the personalized THRR has been calculated, it may be used to determine the appropriate intensity for aerobic activity. To convert the THRR to a 10-second pulse count, simply divide the numbers by 6 (example male's THRR = 24 to 26 per 10 seconds; example female's THRR = 25 to 27 per 10 seconds; see Figure 4.3).

For walking to yield the desired aerobic benefits, it should be done at an intensity level that will produce a heart rate within the desired target heart rate range. Note, however, that in this case more is *not* better. Exceeding your THRR not

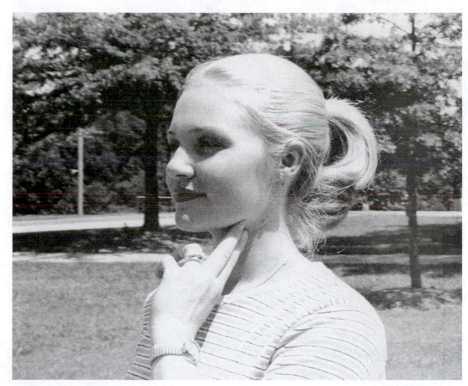

Taking the carotid pulse.

only fails to enhance the effect of the aerobic exercise, but it may also lead to rapid fatigue, causing the exerciser to become discouraged and possibly even call it quits. Forget "no pain, no gain."

When you do flexibility work (stretching), the measure of appropriate intensity is the perception of stretch-tension in the muscle group being stretched. Simply put, the muscle or muscle group should be placed in a stretched position in which you feel a moderate degree of tension (not pain).

The recommended intensity for muscular endurance training may be found in the general rule of thumb that endurance is most effectively gained by exercising against a moderate resistance. When walking, this moderate resistance is supplied by your body weight as the legs carry the body along the walking route.

Duration (How Long Should I Exercise?)

Aerobic activities such as walking should be done within the target heart rate range for a minimum of 20 to 30 minutes, ideally progressing to regular workouts of 30 to 45 minutes for maximum benefit. However, one of the more appealing findings of recent research, especially for people who find 20- to 45-minute workouts difficult to schedule, is that one may benefit from multiple short workouts. For example, walking for 10 minutes three times a day may be as effective as walking once a day for 30 minutes, or three 15-minute walks instead of one 45-minute walk are just as beneficial. Conversely, one may choose to walk longer than 45 minutes, but (from a health fitness perspective) the additional benefits will be minimal.

1. Determine predicted maximum heart rate (PMHR).
   a. Males: PMHR = 210 − 1/2 Your Age
   b. Females: PMHR = 220 − Your Age

   Examples: 20-year-old male (210 − 10 = 200)
   20-year-old female (220 − 20 = 200)

2. Take Resting Heart Rate (RHR).

   Examples: Male RHR = 60
   Female RHR = 80

3. Subtract RHR from PMHR.

   Examples: 20-year-old male with RHR of 60:
   (200 − 60 = 140)

   20-year-old female with RHR of 80:
   (200 − 80 = 120)

4. Multiply answer in #3 by 0.60 and 0.70.

   Examples: Males   (140 × 0.60 = 84 & 140 × 0.70 = 98)
   Female   (120 × 0.60 = 72 & 120 × 0.70 = 84)

5. To get target heart rate range (THRR), add answers in #4 to RHR.

   Examples: Male   (60 + 84 = 144 & 60 + 98 = 158)
   Female   (80 + 72 = 152 & 80 + 84 = 164)
   Male's THRR = 144 to 158 beats/minute
   Female's THRR = 152 to 164 beats/minute

Figure 4.1 Calculating Target Heart Rate Range Worksheet

1. Determine predicted maximum heart rate (PMHR).

   a. Male: 210 − _____ = _____
                    1/2 Your Age   PMHR

   b. Female: 220 − _____ = _____
                         Age   PMHR

2. Take resting heart rate (RHR). _____
                                          RHR

3. Subtract RHR from PMHR.

   _____ − _____ = _____
          PMHR   RHR   Ans. #3

4. Multiply answer in #3 by 0.60 and 0.70.

   a. _____ × 0.60 = _____
            Ans. #3   Ans. #4a

   b. _____ × 0.70 = _____
            Ans. #3   Ans. #4b

5. To get target heart rate range (THRR), add answers in #4 to RHR.

   _____ + _____ = _____
         Ans. #4a   RHR   Lower THR

   _____ + _____ = _____
         Ans. #4b   RHR   Upper THR

Your (THRR) = _____ to _____

Figure 4.2 Calculating Target Heart Rate Range Worksheet

Beats in 10 sec.	=	Beats per minute
10		60
11		66
12		72
13		78
14		84
15		90
16		96
17		102
18		108
19		114
20		120
21		126
22		132
23		138
24		144
25		150
26		156
27		162
28		168
29		174
30		180

Figure 4.3 Heart Rate Conversion Chart

As stated in the earlier discussion of static stretching, the muscle group being stretched should be placed in a stretched position and held there for an appropriate period of time. Though there will be significant variation among individuals, holding a muscle in the statically stretched position for 20 to 30 seconds should produce the desired results. Repeating the 20- to 30-second stretch two or three times is recommended.

The recommended duration for muscular endurance improvement is simply large numbers of muscle contractions, using moderate resistance. During a nice, long walk, the muscles of the legs will contract and relax a thousand or more times.

Frequency (How Often Should I Exercise?)

The most easily answered question in the exercise prescription puzzle is that of exercise frequency. Each general type of exercise—aerobic, flexibility, and muscular endurance—has a rather well-defined recommended frequency. For aerobic improvement, you should walk three to five days per week, while an exercise frequency of two days per week will allow you to maintain your current state of aerobic fitness. An exercise frequency (or infrequency) of one day per week is not recommended, nor is the other extreme, seven days per week, since daily aerobic exercise is associated with a much greater frequency of exercise-related injury.

Flexibility training is one of the few exercise forms that may safely be done everyday. Not only is daily stretching considered safe, but it is highly recommended if you are to maintain and improve your flexibility.

Muscular endurance training can be safely and effectively done three to five days per week. As with the other prescription components, this guideline is the same as that for aerobic improvement, and it fits perfectly with the recommended guidelines for an effective walking program.

"Do It!" Principle

Possibly the most important of all exercise principles is the "Do it!" principle. It has often been said about important issues that when all is said and done, much is said and little is done. This point is too often true when one decides to begin an exercise program. Elaborate plans are made, exercise wear is purchased, but the plan is never converted into action. The "Do it!" principle simply states that for exercise-related health fitness benefits to be realized, you must *do it*—exercise. A wise man once observed, "Words are words, explanations are explanations, promises are promises —but only performance [doing it] is reality." This comment is certainly true of personal exercise programs.

Summary

Walking is an excellent aerobic activity. To receive maximum fitness benefits from walking, however, you should follow some basic exercise principles. Failure to apply sound principles of exercise to your personal fitness walking program not only may reduce the beneficial effects you are trying to achieve but may even result in injury. However, by understanding and correctly utilizing these principles, you will find that walking can be both very beneficial and enjoyable.

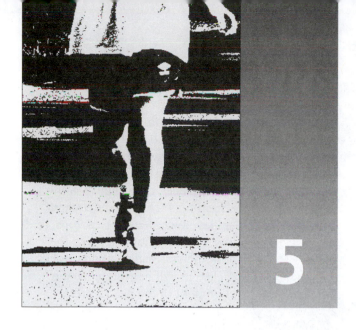

I am a slow walker, but I never walk backwards.

Abraham Lincoln

5

Proper Walking Technique

Whether strolling at an easy 2 to 3 miles per hour or enjoying a brisk fitness walk at 4 miles per hour, it is important to use proper walking technique. Poor posture and mechanics lead to increased stress not only on the lower back but on all the weight-supporting bones, joints, muscles, and ligaments of the lower body. A few simple suggestions may help you avoid many of the common problems experienced by some fitness walkers, such as lower-back pain.

Walking is a skill that you have been practicing for most of your life. The way you walk is as personal and unique as the way you speak. If you are like most people, it will not be necessary to drastically change the way you walk to enjoy the many benefits of fitness walking. For example, walking with the toes pointed slightly outward is quite normal. It is not necessary to force the foot into a perfectly straight alignment. On the other hand, excessive toeing out may, if uncorrected, lead to a variety of physical problems, including chronic leg and back pain. Therefore, to receive maximum enjoyment from your fitness walking program, you must understand and practice proper walking technique.

Body Mechanics

Proper walking technique is not limited to the action of the arms and legs. Good posture, controlled breathing, and relaxation are techniques that also should be mastered and utilized for maximum walking enjoyment.

Posture

Good postural alignment is basic to good walking technique. By maintaining good posture while walking,

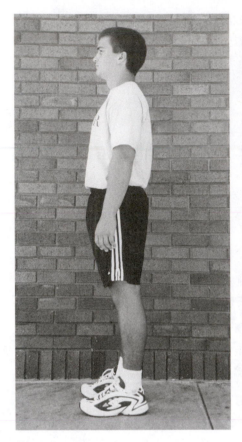

Correct posture.

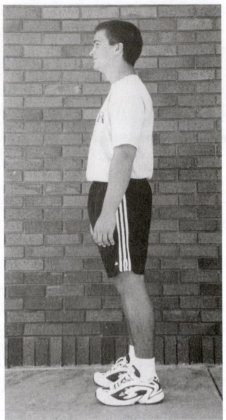

Incorrect posture.

several reasons. First, correct posture gently lifts the ribs away from the lungs, allowing them to function more freely. Second, keeping the body weight evenly distributed over the feet minimizes the stress placed on weight-bearing structures including the arches, ankles, lower legs, knees, hips, and lower back. Finally, keeping the abdomen (stomach) and buttocks tucked in will help stabilize the alignment of the pelvic girdle, reducing stress on the lower back while, at the same time, strengthening and toning the abdominal muscles.

To improve and maintain proper walking posture, the best advice is simply "Hold your head high." It is difficult to have poor posture while holding the head high. Therefore, hold your head up, and good walking posture will tend to follow. Furthermore, there is so much to see that with your head up, you can enjoy the beauty of your surroundings. It would be a shame to miss a lovely sunset because you were looking down at your feet!

Breathing

The second important component of good body mechanics is full, deep, relaxed breathing. Walking is an aerobic activity, so it is important that you provide the body with the oxygen-rich air it needs. Breathing, as simple as it may appear, is often overlooked as an important part of fitness walking.

There are actually two major types of breathing that most people commonly use. *Chest breathing* basically involves the contraction and relaxation of the intercostal (rib) muscles. Somewhat rapid and shallow, it is often associated with stress brought on by fear, anxiety, or the inability to relax. *Abdominal breathing,* on the other hand, is the result

you will find it easier to maintain a consistent stride and breathe fully and normally. Correct posture can also help you avoid the tension and pain in the neck, shoulders, and back that often result from poor posture.

An easy way to check for good postural alignment is, while standing, to draw an imaginary line between the ear and the ankle. This line should pass through the middle of the shoulder, pelvis, hip, and knee. To maintain proper posture when walking, the back should be held erect, with the stomach and buttocks pulled in, the shoulders back, and the head high. This may sound like a tall order, but these positions are all quite natural and can be easily mastered.

By following these simple suggestions, you will notice that you will feel more comfortable for

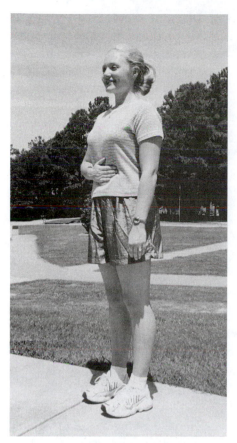

Abdominal breathing can be felt by placing one hand on the abdomen.

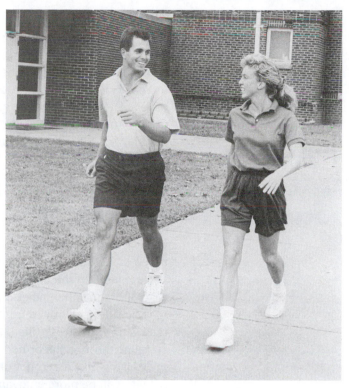

The "talk test"—if you cannot carry on a conversation, you are walking too fast.

of contraction and relaxation of the diaphragm; it is slower, fuller, and more relaxing. To see the difference in these two types of breathing, sit or stand and place one hand on the abdomen (stomach). Abdominal (diaphragmatic) breathing can be felt as the abdomen rises and falls with each breath. Learning to breathe in this manner will enhance relaxation whether resting or walking.

Breathing also offers a convenient way to monitor the appropriateness of your walking pace. When strolling, you should experiment with your breathing rate by using a controlled rate of one inward breath for every four walking strides, followed by one outward breath for four strides. If you can do this comfortably, you are walking at a very relaxed pace. You may find that a good fitness walking pace (as measured by your target heart rate range) requires that you take an inward

breath with every three strides, and likewise with outward breathing. If you find that you must breathe inward and outward at two stride intervals, a check of your heart rate will likely reveal that you are working above your target range, and you may wish to slow down. Learning to breathe in a rhythmic and controlled way enables the lungs and breathing muscles to work most efficiently. With just a little practice, controlled breathing will become a natural part of your body mechanics.

Another way in which breathing may be used as an indicator of your walking pace is commonly called the "talk test." Simply stated, while walking, if you are breathing so rapidly that carrying on a conversation is uncomfortable, you are probably walking too fast. Remember, exercise should be fun.

Relaxation

To some people, the idea of relaxing while exercising may seem like a contradiction. This is because few of us really understand the true nature of relaxation and its importance to our enjoyment of life. Contrary to popular belief, relaxation is not merely sitting back with our feet propped up or lying by the pool on a warm, sunny day. Instead, relaxation is simply functioning physically and mentally with minimal resistance. Therefore, it is quite possible that a highly trained athlete may be more relaxed in the midst of a heavy workout than someone else who may be sitting calmly in front of the television with stress-filled thoughts spiraling through his or her mind.

Walking, like any other physical activity, will be more enjoyable and beneficial when you learn to relax along the way. With that in mind, consider that relaxation entails three basic elements: mechanics, metabolism, and mentality. Let's take a look at each one in more detail.

Mechanics refers to the proper posture and breathing discussed in the previous section. The body will experience difficulty achieving a relaxed state if it must struggle to overcome the negative effects of poor posture and labored breathing. Therefore, the first step in learning to relax is to develop and maintain desirable posture and controlled, relaxed breathing.

Metabolism alludes to the body's fitness level. A person who lacks desirable aerobic fitness will find even light exercise taxing. However, as your fitness improves, so does the ease with which exercise is done. As your body begins to enjoy the many physiological benefits of walking discussed in Chapter 4, you will find that even long, brisk walks will be relaxing.

Mentality simply means that relaxation depends, at least in part, on your state of mind. Good posture, controlled breathing, and a fit body cannot produce a relaxed state if your mind is filled with negative thoughts. Learning to relax means learning to focus your thoughts on the present moment. Walking can put you in touch with the beauty of nature, the fellowship of good friends, and a myriad of other pleasant experiences. Relax, and enjoy them.

Walking Mechanics

Believe it or not, there is a right way and a wrong way to walk. Fitness walking will be more enjoyable, more beneficial, and safer if you learn and utilize good walking mechanics. Above all, however, your individual walking technique should be natural, smooth, relaxed, and enjoyable. Therefore, the following section offers simple, practical advice for developing a walking style that is mechanically sound yet also meets your individual needs.

Arm Action

When you walk or run, the action of the arms will have a direct influence on the length and rate of your stride. While walking, you should hold your arms in a relaxed manner. Many experienced walkers prefer to keep the elbows flexed at approximately 90°, while others find it more comfortable just to allow the arms to extend more naturally at the side—the choice is yours. The hands should form a slightly clinched, though relaxed fist. Allowing the arms to swing naturally back and forth will provide additional power and distance with each stride and will help you maintain your balance.

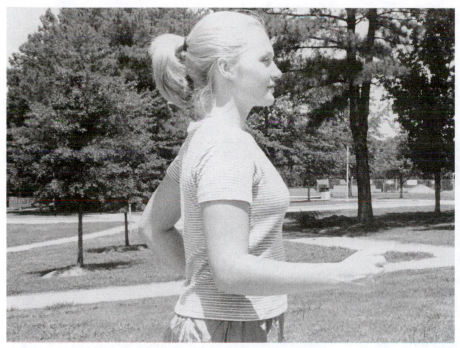

The arms should be relaxed and held at about a 90° angle.

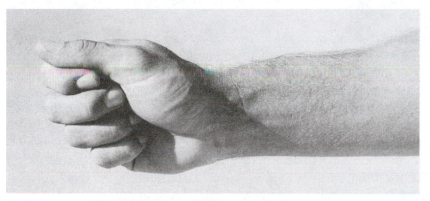

The hands should form a slightly clinched yet relaxed fist.

As noted earlier, the faster you swing your arms, the faster your legs tend to move. Therefore, as you wish to increase your foot speed, a slight increase in the speed of your arm swing will be helpful. Also, vigorous arm action will help increase your heart rate toward the desired target range. The more rhythmic and coordinated the arm swing becomes, the more relaxed and enjoyable walking will be. The best advice is to experiment with arm swing until you find the technique that is most comfortable for you.

Leg Action

Along with proper arm swing, the fitness walker should develop a comfortable, efficient walking stride. Each stride is initiated by a slight forward lean of the body at the ankles. Just at the point when the body begins to feel off balance, the walker steps forward to "catch" the body and prevent falling.

Of utmost importance is the way in which the foot contacts the walking surface. Upon landing, the foot should make contact with the walking surface on the outer edge of the heel. Failure to contact the walking surface correctly may result in injury to the foot, ankle, or both.

Upon impact, the foot should roll smoothly forward with most of the body weight distributed along the outer edge of the foot, transferring the weight to the ball of the foot and then onto the toes for the push-off. A smooth push-off is essential to prevent bouncing. From heel strike to push-off, the foot should remain in contact with the walking surface until the leg is fully extended at the knee. This will help you maintain balance while achieving a smooth, efficient gait.

Pace

As previously discussed, all walking is beneficial, regardless of the type. However, to experience maximum fitness benefits, it is necessary to walk at a fairly brisk pace. Generally, a pace of 3 to 3.5 miles per hour (20 and 17 minutes per mile, respectively) is comfortable for most people. A pace of 3.5 to 4.5 miles per hour (the latter being 13 minutes, 20 seconds per mile) is relatively vigorous, while anything over 4.5 miles per hour is considered really hustling.

To calculate your walking pace, you will need two pieces of

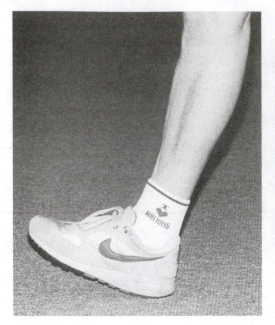

In the heel strike, the foot should make contact with the walking surface on the outside of the heel.

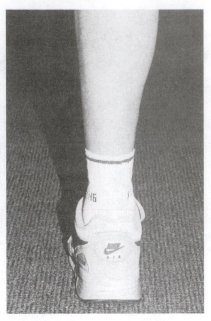

During the stride, most of the body weight should be distributed along the outer edge of the foot.

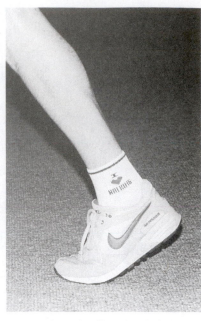

A smooth push-off is essential to prevent bouncing.

information: distance and time walked. The easiest way to calculate the distance you walk is on a pre-measured course such as a ¼-mile track. If you do not have access to a track or premeasured walking trail, drive along your walking route, and use the car's odometer to determine the mileage. Then, see how long it takes you to walk a mile at your chosen walking pace. The following formula may be used to calculate your walking pace:

$$\text{Walking pace (mph)} = \frac{\text{Miles walked} \times 60}{\text{Minutes walked}}$$

For example, if you walk 1 mile in 20 minutes, you are walking at a pace of 3 miles per hour: (1 mile × 60) ÷ 20 minutes = 3 miles per hour. Once you know your walking pace, you can then divide the amount of time you wish to walk by the time required to walk 1 mile at your chosen pace to determine the distance your workout will cover. For example, if you want to walk for 50 minutes at 3 miles per hour (20 minutes per mile), you will need to walk 2.5 miles (50 ÷ 20 = 2.5).

The walking pace you choose should meet your own personal needs and desires. A person with little aerobic endurance (e.g., recovering from illness, overweight, nonexerciser) may find 2 to 2.5 miles per hour (24 to 30 minutes per mile) suitable, while a more fit person will discover that a pace of 3 to 6 miles per hour (10 to 20 minutes per mile) may be necessary to achieve the desired exercise benefits. Most experts consider any pace below 3 miles per hour to be slow, so, if you are in good health, you will probably find that a pace faster than this rate will best meet your needs. Remember, an appropriate fitness walking pace is one that (1) allows you to use controlled breathing and comfortably carry on a conversation, (2) places your exercise heart rate within your individual target heart rate range, and (3) is challenging yet enjoyable.

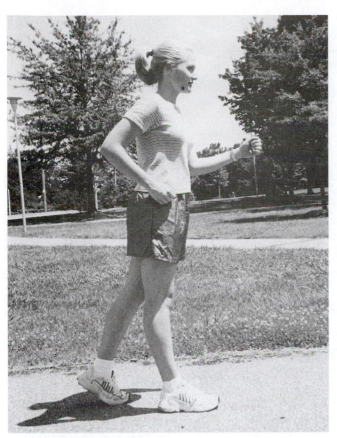

Each stride is initiated by a slight forward lean at the ankles.

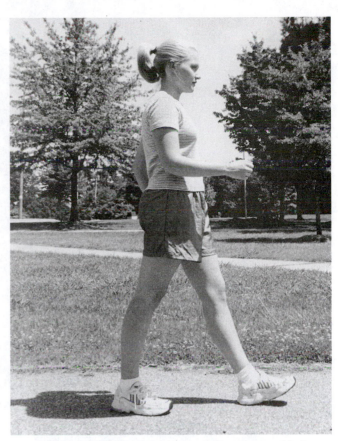

In midstride, the weight should be transferred smoothly from heel strike to push off.

Other Helpful Calculations

In addition to calculating your walking pace, you may find it helpful to use knowledge of your walking pace to make other calculations such as distance walked or time walked. It is really quite simple; as long as you know two of three main fitness walking variables (pace, distance, and time), you can easily calculate the unknown variable. For example, if you know your walking pace and the amount of time you have walked, the estimated distance of your walk is only a brief calculation away.

Walking Distance

Once you have become accustomed to walking at a particular walking pace (e.g., 4 miles per hour), you can then venture out into your neighborhood or a park where the route may not be premeasured for distance. By walking at your chosen pace for a known amount of time (e.g., 30 minutes), the following formula may be used to calculate your distance walked:

$$\text{Miles walked} = \frac{\text{Minutes walked} \times \text{Pace}}{60}$$

In the previous example, in which you have walked at a pace of 4 miles per hour for 30 minutes, your distance walked would be 2 miles.

$$\frac{30 \text{ min.} \times 4 \text{ mph}}{60} = 2 \text{ miles}$$

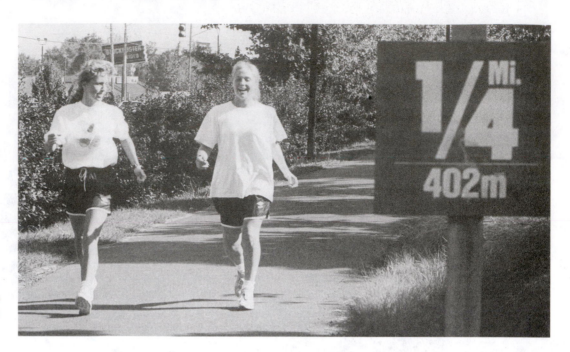

The easiest way to calculate pace is to use a premeasured walking course.

Walking Time

On the other hand, if you know your walking pace and the distance you have walked (or desire to walk), you can easily calculate the time required to walk that distance. The following formula can be used for making this calculation:

$$\text{Walking time} = \frac{\text{Miles walked} \times 60}{\text{Pace}}$$

For example, if you want to walk 3 miles at a pace of 4.5 miles per hour but don't know whether you have enough time to complete the walk and still get to work on time, simply use the formula to find the answer.

$$\frac{3 \text{ miles} \times 60}{4.5 \text{ mph}} = 40 \text{ minutes}$$

If you can do a 40-minute walk and make it to work, great; otherwise, maybe a 30-minute walk would be better. This same formula also comes in handy if you are walking without the benefit of a watch or clock to monitor your time and wish to know how long you have walked (but you must know your pace and distance).

Summary

The more natural the walk, the more likely you are to enjoy the process. Enjoying the process (the walking itself) and not just the product (improved fitness) is really what walking for fun and fitness is all about. It is essential that each walk be worth the time and effort. Too often, we tend to concentrate so much on the end product (improved fitness) that we lose the enjoyment of the process (walking) along the way. Remember, it is the joy of walking that will keep you coming back for more. The fact that you are becoming more physically fit is simply a wonderful bonus. Learning and utilizing proper techniques of posture, breathing, relaxation, and walking mechanics will help you maximize the benefits of your walking program and will also contribute to making your walking more fun.

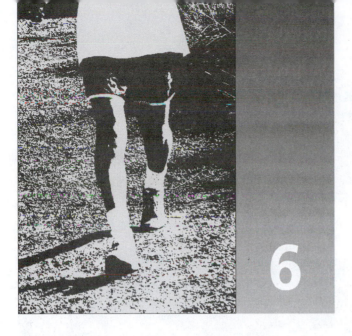

*He who fails to plan,
is planning to fail.*

Author unknown

6

Preparing to Walk

A key factor in the ultimate success of any exercise program is a process that may be called "planning for success." Few people would start out on a vacation trip without some sort of plan for where they were going and the best route to reach their desired destination. Yet, many people begin exercise programs with good intentions but without well-thought-out goals or a plan for accomplishing those goals. The beginning exerciser would do well to heed the advice of the old adage "Plan your work—then work your plan." This chapter will provide some practical suggestions for moving in a positive direction toward literally putting one foot in front of the other, so that walking for fun and fitness becomes an integral part of your daily lifestyle.

Planning for Success

Planning your walking program can be a valuable and enjoyable experience. Careful planning and preparation will enhance your chances of receiving maximum enjoyment and benefits from your walking.

Personal Attitude

It is important that you are convinced that you will be able to stick with your walking program. Your odds of success are much higher if you believe you can! Building confidence (the belief that you can succeed) begins with recognizing and enjoying small successes. As you see yourself succeed with short, easy walks, add more. Also, look around for a role model, someone who started where you are and succeeded at sticking with their exercise program. Such a role model can offer you a sense of personal encouragement. Finally, be realistic about your goals so that you don't become frustrated and give up.

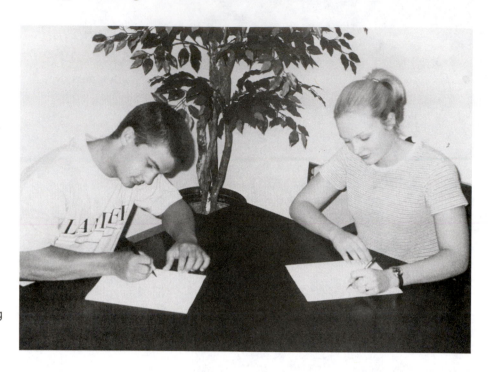

Identify specific walking goals, and put them in writing.

Medical Clearance

Walking is considered a moderate-intensity activity. Therefore, physician clearance is not generally required before starting a fitness walking program. However, it is recommended that men over 40 and women over 50 get physician clearance prior to initiating any vigorous activity (one that would ordinarily cause fatigue in 20 minutes or less). Furthermore, any person, regardless of age, who has known medical problems such as high blood pressure, bone and/or joint problems, or cardiovascular disease should see his or her family physician before starting a walking program.

Physicians generally recommend walking for patients who wish to begin an aerobic exercise program, as well as those recovering from various types of health problems. However, the advisability of using walking or any other form of exercise for rehabilitation depends on the exact nature of the health problem, so it is essential that physician approval be granted.

Goal Setting

Clearly established goals are critical to the success of your walking program, because they provide a means by which you can stay focused on your commitment to a healthier, more enjoyable lifestyle. Even the most dedicated fitness walker will occasionally have to fight the temptation to neglect his or her walking when facing the demands of a busy schedule. By identifying specific goals and putting them in writing, you are much more likely to be consistent in your commitment to achieve those goals.

Goal setting can be a tricky proposition, because, on the one hand, you do not want to select a goal that is so ambitious that achieving it is virtually impossible. If you establish a goal that is unreasonably difficult, you will soon become discouraged and may even want to quit. On the other hand, if your goal is easily attainable with little or no effort, you may become bored and decide the activity is a waste of time. In short, your walking goals should be challenging yet reasonable. Some examples of appropriate long-range goals of a walking program might be as follows:

1. To increase aerobic fitness
2. To walk 200 miles in 6 months
3. To lose 15 pounds

Once you have identified your long-term walking goals, the next step is to map out a plan for accomplishing them. One of the most effective ways of working toward your goals is through the use of short-term performance objectives, which, when accomplished, move you toward the attainment of your goals. As with your long-term goals, short-term performance objectives should be written down. Examples of some short-term performance objectives for attaining the goals stated above include these:

1. To improve aerobic fitness
   a. Walk for 20 minutes, 3 times per week, for 4 weeks
   b. Walk for 30 minutes, 4 times per week, for 4 weeks
   c. Walk for 40 minutes, 5 times per week, on a regular basis
2. To walk 200 miles in 6 months
   a. Walk 2 miles, 3 times per week, for 8 weeks (48 miles)
   b. Walk 3 miles, 3 times per week, for 8 weeks (72 miles)
   c. Walk 3 miles, 4 times per week, for 8 weeks (96 miles)
3. To lose 15 pounds
   a. To walk 20 to 30 minutes, 3 to 5 times per week
   b. To lose 1 pound per week for 15 weeks

Reinforcement Strategy

Another important piece of the "planning for success" puzzle is the development of an effective reinforcement strategy that will keep you moving toward your goals. The most important elements of an effective reinforcement strategy are (1) an "accountability partner" who will support your commitment, not your excuses, and (2) an "accountability plan" that will keep you moving toward your chosen goals. The accountability partner should be someone (friend, roommate, spouse, etc.) who has a copy of your goals and objectives and is willing to hold you accountable for doing what you have said you will do. He or she should be "ruthlessly compassionate" (concerned, but not sympathetic to the point of letting you out of your commitment). The accountability plan is simply an agreed-on time each week when you and your accountability partner will check in with each other to see how you are doing. (See Figures 6.1 and 6.2 and Appendix B.)

Another important aspect of your reinforcement strategy should be positive self-talk. If you are like most people, sometimes you will fail to meet your walking agreement. When this happens, you should resist the temptation to berate yourself but, instead, admit honestly that you did not do what you had planned, restate your commitment, and then *do it!*

Name _____Sally Walker_____   Date __10/1/97_____

Long-term Fitness Goal:

__Improve aerobic fitness_____

_____

Short-term Performance Objectives:

1. __Walk three days each week_____

_____

2. __Walk for at least 30 minutes each day_____

_____

3. __Walk in Target Heart Rate Range for at least 30 minutes each day__

_____

4. _____

_____

Accountability Partner ___Susie Sole_____

Accountability Plan ___Meet each Friday after class_____

_____

___*Sally J. Walker*___   ___*Susie B. Sole*___
Walker's Signature   Partner's Signature

"Ideas are funny little things. They won't work unless you do."
AUTHOR UNKNOWN

Figure 6.1 Personal Walking Accountability Plan

Name _____   Date _____

Long-term Fitness Goal:

_____

_____

Short-term Performance Objectives:

1. _____

   _____

2. _____

   _____

3. _____

   _____

4. _____

   _____

Accountability Partner _____

Accountability Plan _____

_____

_____   _____
        Walker's Signature   Partner's Signature

"Ideas are funny little things. They won't work unless you do."
AUTHOR UNKNOWN

Figure 6.2 Personal Walking Accountability Plan

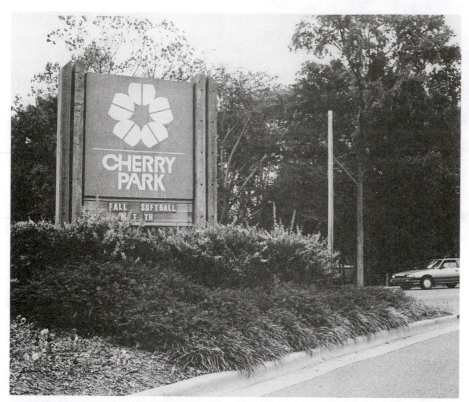

Parks often offer excellent places to walk.

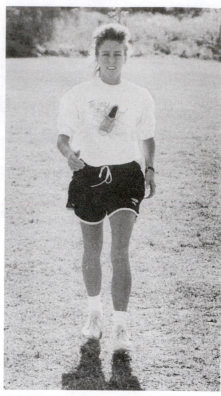

Some people prefer to walk on grass.

Where to Walk

As pointed out in Chapter 2, one of the most appealing features of fitness walking is that it can be done almost anywhere. However, choosing the place or places that best suit your walking needs is critical to the enjoyment and effectiveness of your walking program.

First, you should choose a safe area that is not heavily traveled. A park or track is often a good choice, but many neighborhoods also provide excellent walking routes.

Second, while it is true that you can walk almost anywhere, it is also true that some surfaces are better for walking than others. You will probably find walking on grass or dirt trails more comfortable than concrete sidewalks or streets. The major advantage of the softer walking surfaces is less weight-bearing stress on the feet, ankles, and other body structures, thus resulting in less fatigue and fewer injury problems. However, be aware that when you walk on grass or dirt, poor footing and uneven surfaces may result in ankle sprains. Whether concrete, grass, or dirt, the best advice is to find the surface that best suits your needs.

Third, if you choose to walk along a road, select an area with light traffic, and always walk on the left side facing oncoming vehicles. It is not recommended that you walk after dark unless you have access to a well-lit neighborhood or park, which is virtually traffic-free.

Finally, always use common sense, and be aware of your surroundings. Walking with a friend not only will add enjoyment to walking but also will provide additional security.

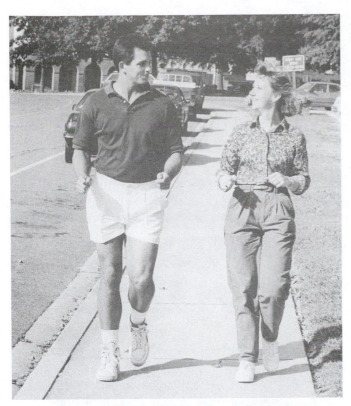

Many walkers enjoy walking on neighborhood sidewalks.

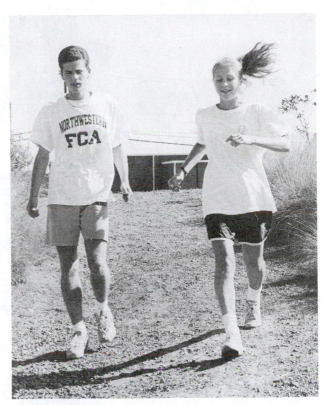

Loose dirt and uneven surfaces may result in poor footing.

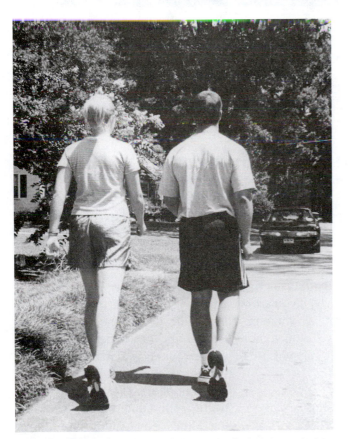

Always walk on the left side of the street, facing oncoming traffic.

When to Walk

One of the most common excuses for not exercising is "I simply do not have the time." In truth, the regular exerciser "has" no more time than the nonexerciser; he or she simply has a commitment to personal fitness and plans exercise time into the daily schedule. The truth is that you make time for those things in your life that are important to you, and what could be more important than enjoying good personal health?

When you choose to walk will depend primarily on your individual daily schedule and personal preference, so look at your options, and go from there. As you plan your walking time, be aware that there will always be people, projects, and other responsibilities that will try to keep you from your commitment. Make walking a priority, and stick with it. The rewards (better health, more energy, reduced stress, etc.) will be worth it.

When planning your walking time, set aside at least 40 to 45 minutes to allow for warm-up, the walk, and cool-down. Since you don't

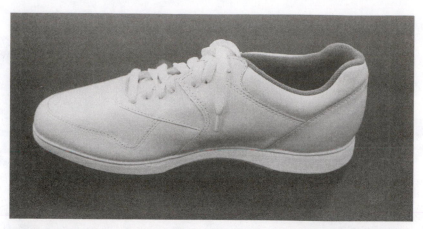

Walking shoe.

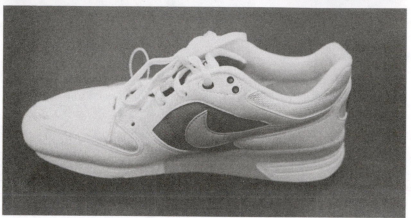

Running shoe.

need a special facility (e.g., gym, pool) for walking, you may be able to simply walk out the door of your house, dorm, or office and immediately step onto your own personal exercise trail. This convenience allows some people to walk on their lunch hour, while others find early morning or late evening the best time to walk.

If walking during your favorite time of the day proves impossible, you may simply have to plan your walk at another time. Early morning may be the only time that fits into your busy schedule. Even if you are not a "morning person," give it a try. The extra energy you get from your morning walk just may compensate for a little lost sleep.

Equipment Selection

Unlike other fitness activities such as swimming, skiing, and bicycling, fitness walking does not require special clothing or equipment. The most important equipment consideration for the walker is a good pair of shoes. Because of our nation's widespread interest in exercise, the variety of exercise footwear available today is literally staggering. Therefore, it is easy to select and purchase an attractive shoe that may not be very appropriate for walking. Several criteria should guide your search for the appropriate walking shoe (Figure 6.3).

The first concern when buying any exercise shoe is finding one that is specifically designed for the activity for which it will be used. In the same way that a marathon runner would not compete in basketball shoes or hiking boots, the walker needs a shoe that is made for walking. Many shoe manufacturers now offer shoes designed specifically for fitness walking. However, this does

Select a shoe that . . . .

1. is activity appropriate (designed for walking)
2. is made of quality materials
3. has a good arch support system
4. is made by a reputable manufacturer
5. fits correctly
6. is well padded and comfortable

Figure 6.3 Criteria for Selecting a Walking Shoe

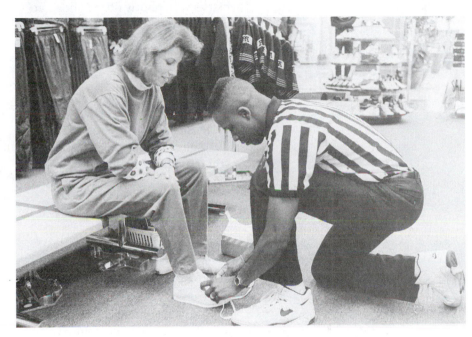

When selecting shoes, consult a footwear professional.

not mean that you will necessarily need to invest in a pair of special walking shoes to enjoy and benefit from your fitness walking program.

The most commonly purchased type of exercise footwear is running shoes. Because of their inherent comfort and attractive design, running shoes are often used for a wide variety of fitness activities, including walking. Running shoes generally have a thick sole, especially under the heel, to provide maximum cushion for the feet while running. However, this elevated design makes the running shoe somewhat unstable, especially if you will be walking on uneven surfaces such as grass or dirt.

If it is true that we get what we pay for, this is especially true when it comes to exercise footwear. Quality exercise shoes are more costly than the less expensive imposters found in some drugstores, discount centers, and even some groceries. A high-quality exercise shoe (1) is made of quality materials, (2) possesses a good arch support system, and (3) is manufactured by a company with a reputation for producing quality fitness footwear. Poor-quality exercise shoes, especially those with little or no arch support, contribute to a host of foot, leg, and back problems, including fallen arches and chronic leg and lower-back pain.

Exercise shoes that fit poorly, even though high-quality, do not provide the comfort or support necessary for enjoyable and productive exercise. The major problems associated with poorly fitting shoes are blisters and other skin irritations on the foot, though shoes that are too small may produce compression and bruising to the toes.

The best advice is to seek the guidance of an exercise footwear professional. Any reputable store that sells running shoes can assist you in finding the right shoe. Shop around until you find the shoe that works best for you.

Clothing Selection

Walking clothing need not be fancy nor expensive. Although colorful, stylish, and lightweight warm-up suits have become a popular part of the American fashion scene, it is not necessary to invest in expensive exercise wear to enjoy and benefit from fitness walking. The clothing you wear for fitness walking should simply be loose fitting (to allow freedom of movement), comfortable, and suitable for existing weather conditions. In warm weather, lightweight clothing that will allow body heat to be dissipated is best. On the other hand, for cold-weather walking, you should wear several layers of clothing to protect you from the cold. Layering allows body heat to be retained in the spaces between the clothing layers and also gives you the option of

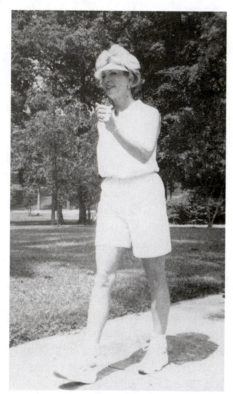

Warm weather walking clothing should be lightweight to promote cooling.

removing individual layers if you become too hot. One of the most important items for cold-weather walking comfort is a cap or other form of head covering, since the body loses much of its heat when the head is uncovered.

Socks should always be worn when walking to avoid the possibility of painful blisters. Cotton socks are best because of their inherent comfort and ability to absorb perspiration efficiently. Women may find that wearing an exercise or sports bra provides added comfort when walking, while men may like the support provided by an athletic supporter.

Optional Items

Other optional walking gear may include such items as a sports watch for timing your walk, a handy fanny pack for carrying small items such as money or personal identification, reflective gear or a flash light for night walking, and/or a walking stick for balance or discouraging an unfriendly animal. None of these items are essential to your walking enjoyment, but you may find them in most sports stores.

One of the more popular accessories among advanced walkers is hand-held weights. Hand weights are generally used in the belief that they will enhance the effect of the workout. Because hand weights are relatively light, they have little effect on caloric expenditure and thus minimal effect on weight loss or management. However, research has shown that using hand weights (with both normal arm swing and exaggerated arm swing) may assist you in reaching your target heart rate range more easily, perhaps at a somewhat slower walking pace than that which would be required without the hand weights.

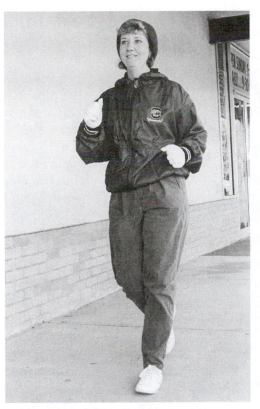

Cold weather walking clothing should be layered to hold in body heat.

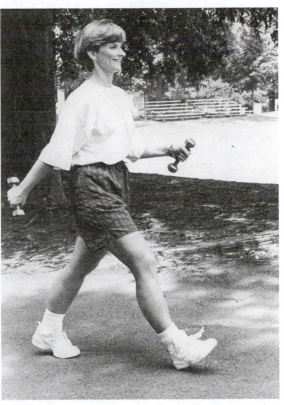

Some walkers use hand weights for a more vigorous workout.

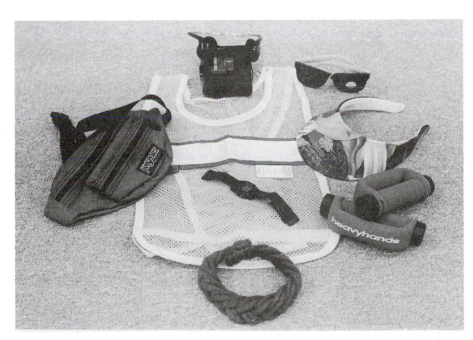

Optional items for the fitness walker.

One of the most recent innovations in fitness walking is "augmented walking," the technique of walking while using striding poles such as those developed and marketed by Tom Rutlin of Exerstrider Products, Inc. Used in much the same way as cross-country ski poles, striding poles offer the experienced walker the same resistance advantages of hand weights, with the added benefits of a more vigorous upper-body (thus total body) workout. Striding poles also provide the walker with added stability and balance.

Hand-held weights and striding poles are not necessary for you to enjoy and benefit from your walking program. However, like other walking accessories, when used properly, they may offer additional benefits and enjoyment.

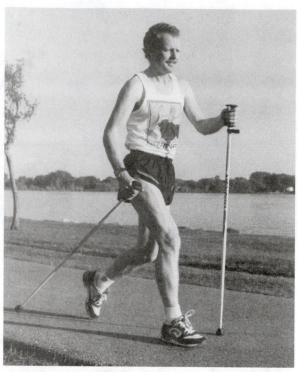

Striding poles are gaining popularity with avid walkers.

Summary

An exciting, enjoyable, and effective walking program does not just happen but is the direct result of careful, thoughtful preparation and the personal commitment to make it work. The best way to "get off on the right foot" with your walking program is to invest time and effort into planning for success. Setting challenging yet realistic goals, developing an effective accountability plan, seeking out convenient and interesting places to walk, planning a time to walk into your daily schedule, and selecting the appropriate shoes and clothing are all important factors in the success and enjoyment of your walking program. Remember, you cannot "work your plan" without first having a plan to work.

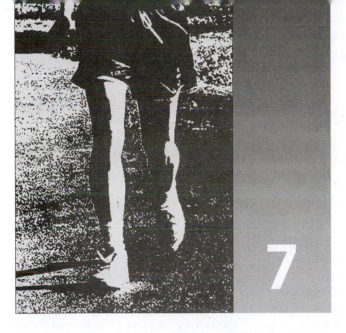

Don't put off for tomorrow what you can do today, for if you enjoy it today, you can do it again tomorrow.

James A. Michener

7

Making the "Do It!" Principle Work for You

Possibly the most important of the exercise principles discussed in Chapter 6 is the "Do It!" principle. Knowing how to walk, when to walk, what to wear, and how fast and how far to walk won't make any difference in your physical health and well-being unless you actually walk! The purpose of this chapter is to do just that—get you on your feet, in your shoes, and out the door.

At this point in your preparation, you should have put your goals in writing and have an accountability partner who is committed to your success. Assuming that this is the first day of your walking program, what do you do first?

Warm-Up and Cool-Down

Every aerobic exercise session (in our case, specifically the fitness walk) should have three distinct phases: (1) warm-up, to get your body prepared for the exercise that lies ahead; (2) fitness walk (the aerobic part of your workout; and (3) cool-down, to allow your body to recover from the workout. All three phases are essential to maximizing the effectiveness and enjoyment of your walking program, as well as lessening your chance of injury.

Warm-Up

Warming up, or getting the body ready for the fitness walk, is one of the most often neglected aspects of a walking program. Many people simply do not see that fitness walking can be very demanding, and they often forego this part of their workout to save time. However, in the case of warm-up there is much truth in the old adage "Haste makes waste" in the form of needless muscle soreness and/or injury.

The warm-up should include two types of activities. First, you should

WARM-UP	W A L K I N G	COOL-DOWN
5–10 minutes	30 minutes or longer	5–10 minutes
• Light Activity • Stretching		• Light Activity • Stretching

Figure 7.1 Daily Workout Plan

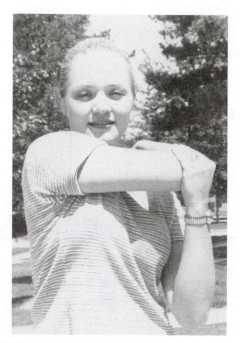

Figure 7.2 Shoulder/Upper Back

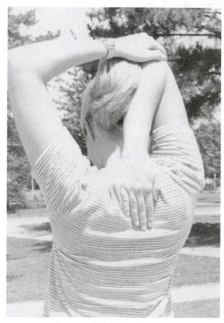

Figure 7.3 Shoulder/Upper Back

do some sort of light, large-muscle activity such as light calisthenics or easy walking while swinging the arms. The purpose of this activity is to warm the muscles and give the cardiovascular system an opportunity to gradually increase its functioning. This part of the warm-up can be completed in about 5 minutes.

Following the muscle-warming activity, you should use static stretching (stretch and hold) to stretch the major muscle groups, thus maximizing the enjoyment of your walk and minimizing the likelihood of exercise-related injury. Static stretching simply involves placing a muscle or muscle group in a stretch position until tension (not pain) is perceived and holding the position without further movement for a period of 20 to 30 seconds. This allows the muscles to relax, thus "loosening" them prior to walking. Ballistic (bouncing) stretching should not be used, since dynamic stretching actually causes reflex contraction of the muscle, which results in tighter rather than looser muscles. Some suggested stretching activities are presented in Figures 7.2 through 7.13.

A light warm-up activity coupled with static stretching can easily be completed in 10 minutes or less and is adequate to increase your heart rate toward your target heart rate range, warm the muscles, and increase short-term flexibility. Static stretching also improves long-term flexibility, decreasing the probability of such problems as chronic muscle soreness, muscle pulls, and even lower-back pain.

Cool-Down

Cool-down is as important as warm-up. Just as the body needs to approach the demands of exercise gradually, it also needs to return to its preexercise state gradually following vigorous exercise. Cool-down activities are similar to those used in warm-up. Immediately following your walk, you should engage in at least 3 to 5 minutes of light activity, such as walking at a leisurely pace or tossing a ball or Frisbee with friends. This activity enables blood that has been directed to exercising muscles during your walk to return to its normal circulatory pattern, rather than "pooling" in the legs, which may cause dizziness or even fainting.

Static stretching following your walk will help reduce the muscle tightness that results from vigorous muscular activity. Also, stretching will improve long-term flexibility and may help prevent or alleviate muscle soreness often experienced by beginning exercisers. Cool-down is also an excellent time to do a few bent-knee abdominal curls to improve and maintain abdominal strength and endurance.

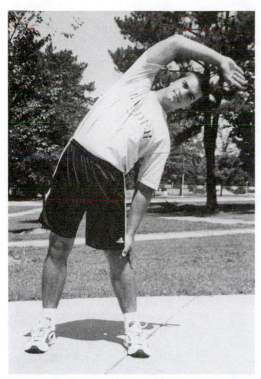

Figure 7.4 Trunk

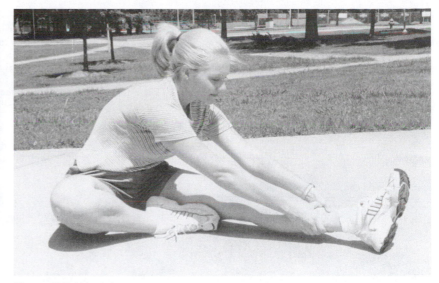

Figure 7.5 Hamstrings

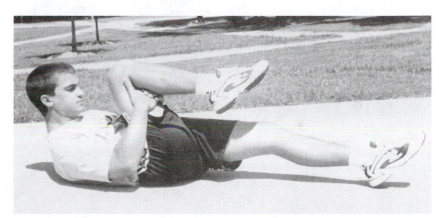

Figure 7.6 Lower Back/Hamstrings

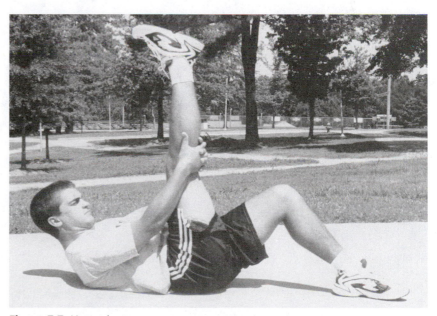

Figure 7.7 Hamstrings

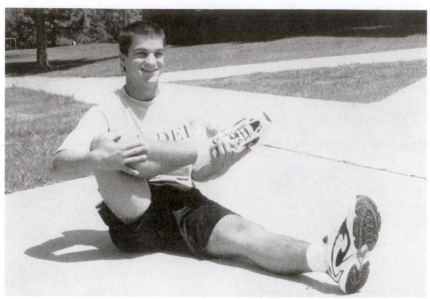

Figure 7.8 Iliotibial Band

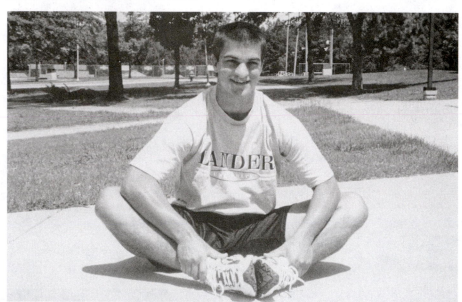

Figure 7.9 Groin

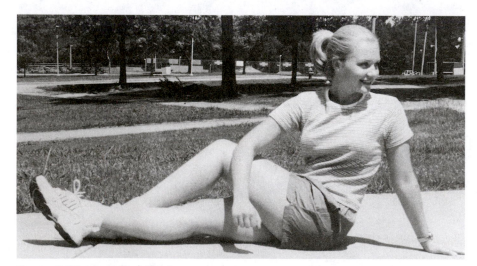

Figure 7.10 Lower Back/Trunk

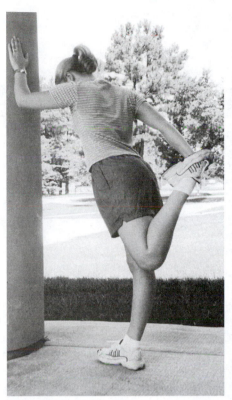
Figure 7.11 Quadriceps

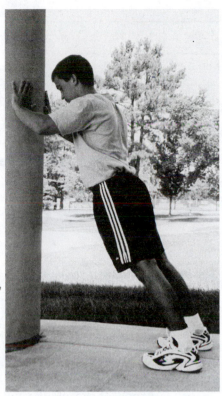
Figure 7.12 Superficial Calves

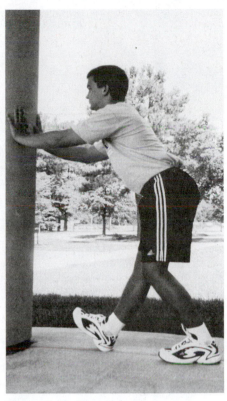
Figure 7.13 Deep Calves

Getting Started

The purpose of your first day's walk is simple—enjoyment. Notice the sky, the trees, the houses, and other walkers. If you are walking with a friend, enjoy the conversation. It may be that exercising and having fun at the same time is a totally new experience for you. That's one of the great things about walking—it enables you to get fit and have fun doing it.

It is important that you start out gradually, especially if you are a beginner or have not exercised for a while. Your first walk should only be about 10 to 15 minutes. Before you start, check your pulse and remind yourself of the pulse count that represents your target heart rate range. About halfway through your walk, stop and check your pulse to see if you are in your target range. If you are below your range, you may want to quicken the pace. Note that increasing your pace by using shorter and quicker strides will elevate the heart rate more effectively than using longer strides. If you are above your range, you may wish to slow the pace a bit. You may find that, in the early stages of your walking program, you are more comfortable when your heart rate is in the lower end of your target range. As you increase your endurance, you may want to work toward the upper end of your target range.

Monitoring your pulse rate periodically is very important, especially when you are just starting your program. However, as you become accustomed to "what it feels like" to be in your target range, you will probably find it unnecessary to check you pulse during each walk.

Week	1	2	3	4	5	6
Minutes	10–15	15	20	25	30	30
Days	3	4–5	3	4–5	3	4–5

* After 6 weeks, walk a minimum of 30 minutes 3–5 times per week. Ideally, you should continue to progress until you are walking 4–5 days per week, for 45–60 minutes per day at a pace of 3 miles per hour or faster.

FIGURE 7.14 Walking Starter Program

The important thing is to listen to your body, and remember that it is neither necessary nor wise to walk at an uncomfortably fast pace. Doing so stresses the cardiovascular system more than is necessary for aerobic conditioning, and it simply doesn't feel good. At the end of your walk, check your pulse again, then once more after cool-down. If you have walked at an appropriate pace, your heart rate should be less than 100 beats per minute (16 to 17 beats for 10 seconds) following a 10-minute cool-down.

A recommended 6-week starter program is presented in Figure 7.14. Following this program will enable you to increase your walking pace and distance gradually and safely.

Sticking With It

People often start a regular exercise program, only to find it difficult to stick with it. It's not that they don't want to exercise regularly or that they don't recognize the benefits of personal fitness. Even the most enjoyable exercise program may get pushed aside when waning interest or other commitments begin to take their toll. The key to sticking with your walking program is to identify resources that you can use to reinforce your commitment and make walking even more fun and rewarding.

Your Accountability Plan

Your accountability plan may be the single most important factor in helping you keep your commitment to a healthier lifestyle and accomplishing your fitness goals. Telling someone else what you are going to do, rather than keeping it a secret, puts your commitment on a different level. Also, there will likely come a time when you may decide to quit or take an extended break from your exercise program. At this time, your accountability partner can offer the support necessary to put you back in touch with your original commitment.

Your accountability partner need not be your best friend, although that may be fine if he or she is someone who will not accept your excuses for not keeping your commitment to walking. The best partner is one who is willing to be "ruthlessly compassionate," which means that he or she will be understanding without being overly sympathetic. Your accountability partner should be someone who will provide support and encouragement; not someone who will let you off too easily.

It is easy to lose sight of your commitment when the hectic pace of everyday life pulls you in so many directions. However, it is because we all live such busy lives that a fitness program, such as walking, is so essential to help us stay physically able to meet the many demands that we face every day.

Your accountability plan is simply an agreement to touch base with your accountability partner on a regularly scheduled basis. This can be done by e-mail, over the telephone, or in person. Choose a designated time each week, and stick to your agreement.

It is essential that you honestly convey your progress to your partner and that you do so quickly and without a lot of unnecessary explanation as to why you did or did not accomplish your weekly goal. This is meant to be a "reporting-in" time, rather than a time of social conversation.

Respect the fact that your partner also has a busy schedule in addition to supporting you and your commitment. Limit your appointment to a few minutes, but make the most of the time you have.

A typical telephone conversation between you and your accountability partner may be something like this: (You) "Hi, Chris. This is _____. Just wanted you to know that I walked three times this week for 30 minutes each time." (AP) "That's great! You are right on schedule. Keep up the good work, and check in next week." Or sometimes your conversation may go something like this: (You) "Hello, Kelly. This is _____. It's really been a rough week. I only walked one time for about 30 minutes."

(AP) "That's tough, but we both knew there would be weeks like that. What does next week look like?" (You) "It's hard to say because of all the work I have ahead of me." (AP) "OK. Let's look at your schedule. Can you get up 30 minutes earlier or find some time between classes? This is just as important as eating and sleeping, so what can you do to make it work?" (You) "I will walk three times next week for 30 minutes. I know—I usually go back to the dorm between chemistry class and my afternoon psychology class. I will work in a walk then." (AP) "Good! I know you can do it. Let me hear from you on Friday."

Notice that there is no criticism for not keeping your agreement, but neither does the accountability partner offer sympathy or agreement that you were too busy to walk three times as planned. The accountability partner is in a position to be more objective, and he or she can offer you some space to look at options you may not otherwise consider. A good accountability partner can be your most valuable asset. Make your accountability plan and accountability partner work to your advantage.

Charting Your Progress

One of the easiest and most effective ways to monitor the progress of your walking program is to put it in writing by keeping a daily log. Your walking log can be an effective source of motivation as well as a convenient method of evaluating the success of your accountability plan (see Figures 7.15 and 7.16 and Appendix C).

Name <u>Robert Notquite Fittenuff</u>   Week # _____

DATE	TIME	DISTANCE	PACE	CALORIES	COMMENTS
9/21	00:30	2.0	4.0	200	The walk was great. I played some memory games.
9/22	00:35	2.5	4.3	265	Felt tired. Think I upped my pace too soon.
9/24	00:35	2.3	3.9	220	Day off helped. Felt like I had more energy today.
9/25	00:40	2.5	3.75	310	Walked with a friend, and really enjoyed it.
9/27	00:30	2.0	4.0	200	4.0 mph feels good to me & gets my HR up to THR
Total	2:50	12.3	**XX**	1195	

Figure 7.15 Walking Log

Name _____   Week # _____

Date	Time	Distance	Pace	Calories	Comments
Total			**XX**		

Figure 7.16 Walking Log

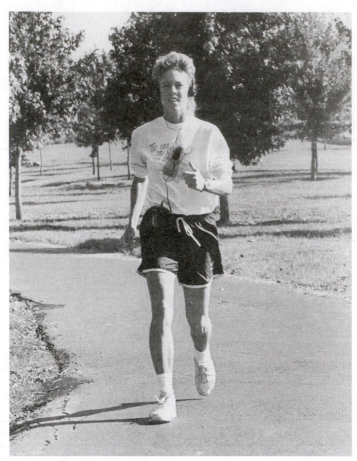

Listening to your favorite music or a walking tape can add to your walking enjoyment.

Ideas and Games Just for Fun

Once your walking program has become an established part of your weekly routine, you may wish to experiment with some innovative ideas and games that other walkers have found to be fun. Some of these games may remind you of ones you played as a child, only with a walking twist. Try them, enjoy them, and use them to add enjoyment to your walking.

Ideas/Games for One

Some ideas and games can be used while walking alone. Try some of the following, and then make up some of your own.

Counting Games

When you were a child, you probably played counting games to pass the hours while traveling in the car. As you walk, try counting the number of

- people you see walking a dog,
- couples you pass,
- bicyclists,
- red (or any color) cars,
- airplanes,
- girls who have ponytails, or
- boys who are wearing caps/hats.

Nature Games

Depending on the season and the section of the country in which you live, try

- identifying five different types of trees,
- noticing which way the wind is blowing,
- picking out animal shapes in the clouds, or
- seeing how may colors you can count in the sunset or sunrise.

Music Games

This type is a personal favorite. Using a radio, tape player, or CD player, listen to your favorite songs or try an aerobic walking tape or CD if you want to speed up your pace. See Chapter 11 for suggested tapes.

Memory Games

As you walk, try to

- name all 50 states and their capital cities,
- remember the first names of all your cousins,
- remember all your teachers beginning with first grade,

- try to remember every person you ever kissed (yes, including Aunt Hazel), or
- recall as many birthdays as you can.

Study Games

If you must memorize lists, names, or dates, walking provides a nice, peaceful opportunity for some enjoyable studying. Keep in mind, however, that walking is your own personal haven from stress, so don't let this become a stressful game.

Fantasy Games

Although you may be walking in familiar surroundings, that doesn't mean that you can't let your mind wander to new and exciting places/events. Some fun activities may include these:

- planning a vacation trip, and money is no object;
- visualizing your dream house—where it will be, what it might look like;
- fantasizing about how you would spend the money if you really did win the grand prize on *Who Wants to Be a Millionaire?* or the Publishers' Clearinghouse Sweepstakes;
- contemplating what you might do if you had three wishes.

Ideas/Games for Groups

Many walkers prefer walking with a friend or group of friends to walking alone. Others find that walking with a friend or group of friends simply adds variety to their walking program. When you walk with others, try one of the following games or take turns making up your own.

Conversation Games

When two or more people walk together, conversation can be turned into a game. Two rules should be used to guide conversation games. First, everyone should remember the "talk test" (see Chapter 5), and if the walking pace makes conversation uncomfortable, slow down. Second, limit the conversation game to one topic per walk, and you may be surprised how much can be said on one subject. Suggested topics include these:

- My idea of the perfect date is . . . .
- My most embarrassing moment was . . . .
- My favorite restaurant is . . . because . . . .
- The place I would like to visit most is . . . .
- The most interesting place I have been is . . . .
- The most famous person I have ever met is . . . .
- The person I would most like to meet is . . . .

Interaction Games

Similar to conversation games, interaction games are suggested for groups in which the members may not know each other well, such as fitness classes and walking clubs. Have everybody get into groups of three or more. While on the walk, each member of the group must find out specific things about other people in their group, such as

- favorite foods;
- preferred brand of toothpaste, shampoo, and so forth;
- number of brothers and sisters;
- favorite TV show, movie, and so forth; and

■ what I want to be when I grow up. (This one is not just for children—many adults are still deciding!)

Walking Poker

This is a variation of the familiar card game. Prior to the walk, one member of the group is designated the dealer and is given a deck of standard playing cards. The dealer shuffles the cards and deals one card to each walker. Without disclosing their card, the group members begin their walk. At the first pulse rate check stop, each group member is dealt a second card. A third card is dealt to each group member at the next pulse rate check stop, and a fourth at the next. Each group member receives a fifth card at the conclusion of the walk, and the one with the best poker hand is the winner. To make the game even more interesting, the group members may agree in advance to "chip in" and buy the winner a cone of his or her favorite frozen yogurt, a diet soft drink, or some other fun reward.

Ideas/Games for Clubs

While some walkers prefer to walk alone, and others enjoy walking with a partner or a small, casual group, some more formal walking groups such as walking clubs or classes enjoy making their walking program a team effort. This approach not only encourages individual walking but uses collective effort as an effective motivation technique.

Geography Games

The group plans an imaginary trip. It may be across the nation, across Europe, or any itinerary that interests the group. By consulting with a travel agent, the exact mileage from one city to the next along the way can be determined. Each member of the group turns in his or her walking mileage on a weekly basis, and the total mileage walked by the entire group is recorded on a chart. A weekly progress report can be used to inform the group exactly where they are along the trip route. Various members of the group can be enlisted to prepare a brief report on cities or points of interest along the route to be shared with the entire group at the appropriate time. When the destination is reached, plan a party to celebrate. One such group "walked" from South Carolina to Hawaii and then celebrated with a luau. Geography games can be not only fun and motivational but educational as well.

Walk to a Vacation Destination

First, determine how much money it would cost for two people to go to the vacation destination of choice (including one night's lodging and meals). Divide the total cost among the number of participants in the game, and have each person contribute his or her share. Determine the exact mileage to the vacation destination of choice, and establish that as your mileage goal. Each group member then turns in his or her walking mileage on a daily basis. The first person to reach the mileage goal wins the prize money for the "minivacation" trip. A motel or hotel at the vacation destination may even agree to donate a night's lodging in return for the publicity the event will provide.

Money Games

For some walkers, money is the most effective motivation. Mileage-based money games are easy to create and often very effective. For example, have each group member chip in an agreed-on amount of money (e.g., $1, $5, etc.) or solicit the support of a corporate sponsor from the local community. The first person to walk a total of 100 miles (or any goal selected by the group) wins the cash.

Another approach is to create a time-based money game. The group agrees on a time frame—say, 6 months. At the end of 6 months, the person who has walked the most miles wins the cash. Some groups prefer to have a first-, second-, and third-place prize rather than one person winning all the money.

For some people, these ideas/ games may not offer much appeal. However, if you enjoy talking and playing games or are simply interested in making a fun activity like walking even more enjoyable, then these should provide you with some food for thought. They are certainly not necessary to enjoy walking, but, from personal experience, they can provide an added boost to your walking fun.

Incentives and Rewards

Can you remember how good it felt to get an A for a paper on which you worked really hard? Maybe you can recall the first paycheck you ever received or your first allowance for doing jobs around the house. These were simply rewards for doing a good job and also an incentive to continue doing a good job. That strategy worked when you were 10 years old, and it can work just as well when you are 20, 30, or 99. The difference is that now you will be the one planning the rewards for yourself, rewards that will recognize the achievement of certain goals along the way to accomplishing your ultimate goal—improved aerobic fitness.

You should choose rewards that are special, but not necessarily expensive. Some examples of inexpensive rewards for keeping your commitment for the first 3 weeks might be

- a new pair of walking socks,
- a sweat band or wrist band,
- a fanny pack, or
- your favorite yogurt.

After keeping your commitment for 6 weeks, treat yourself to

- a night out on the town,
- a long-distance phone call to someone really special, or
- dinner at your favorite restaurant.

After 12 weeks, treat yourself to

- a new CD or cassette tape,
- a new outfit, or
- a new sports watch.

When you reach a special milestone, such as losing the desired amount of weight or maintaining a walking program for 1 year:

- how about a special trip or
- a new pair of walking shoes?

Just remember that rewards and incentives serve two purposes. They represent a "pat on the back" for keeping your commitment, and they provide motivation for keeping on. Make the most of the reward/incentive idea by choosing something for which you are willing to work hard. The ideas mentioned, although popular with many fitness walkers, may not appeal to you. Make your own list, and feel free to change it. However you choose to use rewards and incentives, make them work for you.

Summary

The most important part of any walking program is doing it—walking. To receive the many benefits that walking has to offer, you must put your plan into action. Every walk should begin with a warm-up and end with a cool-down to give your body an opportunity to adjust gradually to the exercise demands and minimize the chance of exercise-related injury. Once you have begun your walking program, the challenge is to stick with it. You will find that a good accountability partner will be an invaluable resource in helping you keep your commitment to walking, and the number and variety of activities for keeping the fun in your walking are endless.

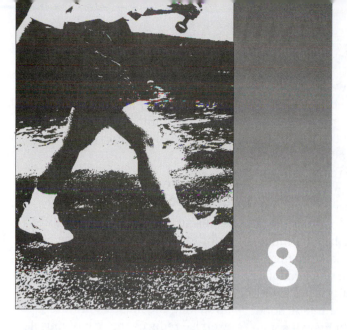

A man too busy to take care of his body is like a mechanic too busy to take care of his tools.
Spanish proverb

8

Prevention and Care of Injuries

Fitness walking offers numerous health-related benefits, and it is among the safest of all types of exercise. However, it is not a risk-free activity. Any time the body is put into motion, the possibility exists of injury or illness either directly or indirectly related to the exercise program itself. Most such injuries and illnesses are preventable if you simply follow a few guidelines based on common sense. When an unavoidable injury or illness does occur, its severity may be dramatically reduced if it is cared for promptly and properly. Therefore, this chapter presents a systematic plan for preventing and caring for exercise-related injuries and illness. The information contained in this section is not intended to provide medical advice, and it should not be substituted for a physician's care when such care is warranted.

Injury Prevention

A familiar adage states, "An ounce of prevention is worth a pound of cure." While somewhat simplistic, this statement is nevertheless very true with respect to exercise-related injury and illness. As will be discussed later, caring for an injury is often a time-consuming and complicated process, not to mention frustrating if you must discontinue your walking program while healing takes place. Therefore, the key to enjoying injury-free fitness walking is to prevent injuries and illness from occurring in the first place.

Following the Principles of Exercise

The injury prevention process begins with a thorough knowledge and application of the basic principles of exercise (see Chapter 4). The overzealous fitness walker may choose to ignore the principle of progression by suddenly increasing the distance he or she walks or the pace at which the walking is done, only to find that the results are not faster gains but chronic fatigue, soreness, and/or pain.

Likewise, failure to follow the recommended guidelines for intensity, duration, and frequency may produce one or more of a host of exercise-related injuries. The safest exercise is the exercise that is done correctly and in keeping with sound scientific principles.

Selection of Proper Equipment

Carefully selected and properly fitted exercise equipment can enhance the enjoyment of exercise. However, inappropriate, poor-quality, and ill-fitting equipment can actually result in injury. Probably the most important single piece of equipment for any type of exercise is the footwear. Since the feet provide the major support for the body weight while walking, the selection of good-fitting, comfortable, supportive shoes is of utmost importance in preventing foot, ankle, leg, knee, hip, and lower-back injuries (see Chapter 6).

In addition to footwear, the selection of proper walking clothing is also important in injury and illness prevention. Walking clothing should be comfortable, relatively loose fitting, and made of materials that will allow the body to rid itself of the heat produced by exercise. Wearing heat-trapping clothing is a major contributing factor to heat illness, especially during the summer months. Such devices as rubber suits and "sauna suits" have become popular among those trying to lose weight. While exercising in such garments will result in the loss of body water, and therefore weight,

this weight loss is short term and potentially very dangerous. Heat-trapping clothing should never be worn in an attempt to lose weight.

Warming Up and Cooling Down

As discussed earlier, warming up prior to walking prepares the body for the impending demands of the exercise itself. Most sports medicine experts agree that warming and stretching the muscles prior to exercise reduces the risk of muscle pulls (strains) and exercise-related muscle soreness.

The injury prevention benefits of cool-down are similar, since muscles that have been subjected to vigorous exercise often tend to tighten and must be stretched if optimal flexibility is to be maintained. Failure to maintain optimal flexibility may result in such exercise-related injuries as muscle pulls, chronic muscle soreness, chronic lower-leg pain (often referred to as *shin splints*), and even ankle sprains.

Knowing When to Stop Exercising

In most cases, when walking is done correctly, the body responds positively to the demands placed on it. However, if, while walking, any of the following symptoms should appear, you should stop immediately and seek professional advice:

1. Chest pain
2. Nausea, dizziness, fainting, vomiting, and the like
3. Significant headache
4. Excessive shortness of breath
5. Excessive fatigue
6. Musculoskeletal pain

These symptoms may indicate that the body is not responding

positively to the exercise, and you should be evaluated prior to returning to your walking program. Failure to heed the body's "warnings" may result in injury or illness.

Knowing When Not to Exercise

There are times when it is simply not advisable to exercise. Among these are when (1) you are ill, (2) you are injured, and (3) it is extremely hot and humid.

When your body is suffering from illness (even a common cold), it generally will not respond positively to exercise. In fact, the demands of exercise may actually complicate the illness. Though a common belief, "sweating out a fever" is a very unwise and potentially dangerous practice.

Walking when you are injured is simply not very smart. As will be discussed later, injuries generally respond favorably to rest, especially during the early stages of healing. Exercising while injured may seem like the "macho" thing to do, but the result will only be a prolonged time of healing and possibly even further damage to the injured body part. The lone exception to this recommendation is the use of physician-recommended exercise for the purpose of injury rehabilitation.

The dangers of exercising in extreme heat and humidity are discussed in later sections.

Injury Care

Unfortunately, not all exercise-related injury and illness can be prevented. When injury or illness does occur, it is important that the problem be managed properly to avoid complicating the situation. Generally, the process of exercise-related injury and illness self-care

may be summarized in the following manner:

1. Act promptly. (Don't wait until later.)
2. Act conservatively. (When in doubt, consult a physician.)
3. Act correctly. (Follow accepted first aid and self-care guidelines.)

The most common walking-related injuries and illnesses are (1) musculoskeletal injuries such as muscle strains ("pulls"), ankle sprains, and chronic muscle soreness; (2) blisters and other skin inflammations; and (3) heat illness.

Musculoskeletal Injuries

Research indicates more than 50% of all exercise-related injuries involve the muscles, bones, joints, and related structures. Although it is beyond the scope of this book to present a detailed plan for each individual type of musculoskeletal injury, most musculoskeletal injuries respond best to PRICE—not the cost of your walking shoes or favorite CD, but an injury care regimen consisting of **p**rotection, **r**est, **i**ce, **c**ompression, and **e**levation.

Protection against further injury is the first step in self-care for common musculoskeletal injuries. All too often, when one turns an ankle or pulls a muscle, the tendency is immediately to try to walk on or use the injured joint/muscle. While it may be possible to walk on a recently hurt ankle or use an injured muscle, this does not indicate that the injury does not need proper care. In fact, walking and/or other types of movement of a recently injured joint or muscle may actually increase the severity of the injury and delay healing. When a muscle,

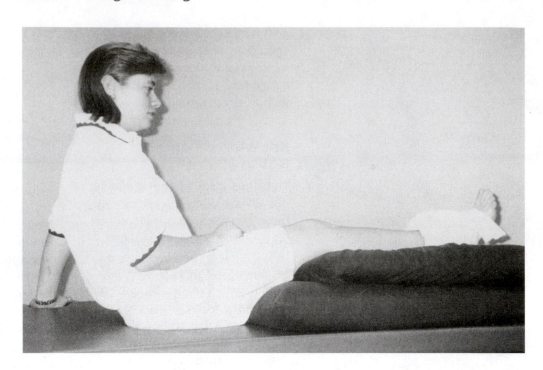

PRICE = **P**rotection, **r**est, **i**ce, **c**ompression, and **e**levation.

bone, or joint injury occurs, protect the hurt area from further trauma by avoiding unnecessary movement or use of the injured body part.

Rest simply means to stop using the injured body part until it has had the opportunity to recover from the initial trauma of the injury. This rest may be as brief as 24 hours for a mild injury or as long as several days or even weeks for a more serious one, and it may require the use of a sling, crutches, or simply rest.

Ice refers to the use of ice, ice water, or cold compresses to retard swelling and promote healing. The most common forms of ice application include (1) placing a cold, wet cloth on the injury, covering it with an ice bag or plastic bag filled with ice, and securing it in place with an elastic wrap; and (2) submerging the injured body part in an ice water bath for 15 to 20 minutes. For maximum benefit, ice treatments should be repeated several times throughout the day, but for no longer than 20 minutes at any one time.

Compression is the use of an elastic wrap (i.e., as an Ace bandage) to control swelling. Compression should be used during the post-acute stage (for several days following the injury) at all times when ice treatments are not in progress. The lone exception to this recommendation is that compression wraps should not be worn at night while sleeping.

Elevation simply means placing the injured body part in an elevated or raised posture, by placing a pillow under the injured body part, for example. This facilitates blood flow away from the injury site and reduces the possibility of swelling that may delay healing. Elevation should be used throughout the postacute stage.

Musculoskeletal self-care should be used only when you have no reason to suspect a more serious injury such as fracture or dislocation. In the event that you do suspect such injury or the injury fails to respond positively to normal self-care procedures, you should consult a physician at once.

Common Walking-Related Musculoskeletal Injuries

When walking, the primary weight-supporting structures are the feet. Therefore, foot injuries are the most common musculoskeletal injuries among fitness walkers.

Each foot has two major arch systems. The *transverse arch* spans the ball of the foot laterally and cushions the force produced by the body weight during the push-off phase of each stride. The *longitudinal arch* spans the midfoot from the anterior portion of the heel to the ball of the foot, and it acts as the body's main weight-supporting system throughout the transfer of weight from heel strike to push-off. Because of the repeated stress placed on these arches during walking, jogging, and running, they must be adequately supported to avoid their breakdown and painful injury to the foot, ankle, lower leg, and possibly other weight-supporting joints.

Metatarsalgia

Pain, and fatigue along the ball of the foot, often accompanied by chronic calluses may be signs of *metatarsalgia,* a chronic inflammation of the transverse arch. Although PRICE care may provide symptomatic relief, long-term relief usually requires better transverse arch support in your walking shoes. Professional advice (from an athletic trainer, fitness professional, exercise footwear specialist, podiatrist, or physician) should be sought concerning the best type of support for you.

Plantar Fasciitis

Another common injury among fitness walkers is *plantar fasciitis,* an inflammation of the supportive connective tissue (plantar fascia) spanning the sole of the foot from the heel to the base of the toes. Sharp pain just anterior to the heel, which is often most noticeable when you first step out of bed in the morning, may indicate plantar fasciitis. Proper arch-supporting shoes with flexible soles (rigid soles will aggravate this problem) and PRICE care are recommended. Also, heating the painful area (heating pad, hot water towel, etc.) prior to walking and applying ice for 15 to 20 minutes immediately following your walk may provide effective pain relief. As with any injury, if these simple suggestions fail to resolve the problem, you should seek professional advice.

Chronic Lower-Leg Pain

Most arch problems involve the longitudinal arch and may cause pain and fatigue along the arch and/or shin splint–type pain along the anterior surface of the shin. A combination of enhanced arch support (with new shoes, insoles, custom orthotics, etc.), PRICE care, and calf stretching (see Chapter 7) will usually result in significant pain relief. If, however, pain does not resolve, or shin pain is accompanied by numbness on the top of the foot and/or weakness when you attempt to use the muscles of the foot to pull the foot and toes up, a physician should be consulted to determine the underlying cause of the injury.

Most foot and leg pain associated with fitness walking will respond positively to the application of sound walking mechanics; the use of good-quality, supportive shoes; the maintenance of desirable flexibility through daily stretching; and the conservative self-care suggestions presented here. Unresolved musculoskeletal pain or discomfort,

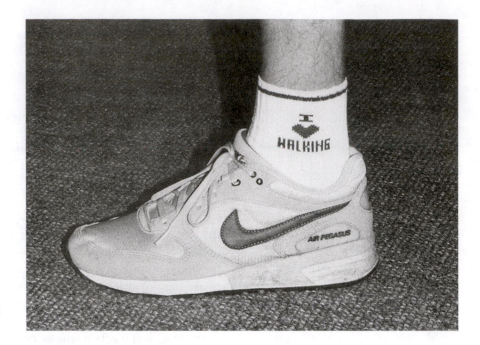

Always wear socks when walking to protect against blisters.

however, should receive prompt medical attention.

Common Walking-Related Skin Conditions

Blisters

Among the most common and most painful of all walking-related injuries is the common blister. Its causes are as varied as the many body parts it may affect, though the common factor in the formation of all blisters is friction. The first step in blister prevention and care is to reduce the friction on blister-prone body parts. Simply stated, socks should be worn when walking, shoes with worn and rough liners should be replaced, and lubricant (e.g., petroleum jelly), powder, or an adhesive bandage (i.e., a Band-Aid) should be used to prevent "hot spots" (preblister friction irritation sites) from becoming full-fledged blisters.

The key in caring for blisters is to keep them intact if at all possible, since a ruptured blister provides an excellent opportunity for infection. Most blisters may be kept intact by placing a felt or foam rubber doughnut (a piece of felt or foam with a hole the size of the blister cut in it) over the blister, and securing it in place with tape. This protects the blister from pressure that may cause it to rupture. The second step is to attempt to get the blister to reabsorb or "go down." Removing the pressure by use of a doughnut will usually allow the blister to reabsorb, but the process may be enhanced by soaking the blister in ice water several times a day. Once the fluid from the blister has been reabsorbed, continued use of the doughnut for a few days will allow the blister to heal, and no further care should be necessary. Should a blister rupture, clean it carefully, treat with an antiseptic spray or ointment, cover with a sterile dressing, and protect from infection until healed.

Calluses

A common problem among fitness walkers is the existence of chronic

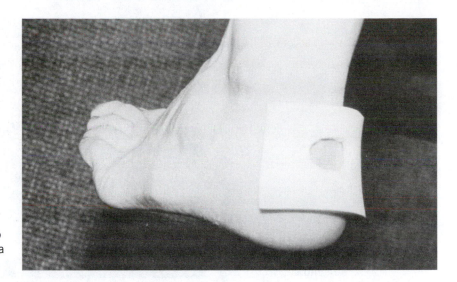

One of the best ways to protect a blister is with a foam rubber doughnut.

friction leading to the formation of calluses. A *callus* is an area of thickened skin that, if not cared for properly, may become hardened and painful. The initial step in caring for calluses is similar to that for blisters —identify the cause, and remedy it. This may require the assistance of an exercise footwear professional in the case of foot calluses.

To soften calluses, the area may be soaked daily in hot water several times a day, followed by rubbing lotion into the callused skin. If calluses remain painful or appear to have a collection of blood beneath them, a physician should be consulted.

Heat Illness

One of the most dangerous of exercise-related conditions is heat stress or heat illness. Heat illness is the result of the body's inability to adjust to conditions of high temperature and humidity.

Preventing Heat Illness

The most prudent way to approach heat illness is to prevent it from occurring in the first place. This simply requires using common sense, by (1) not exercising outdoors when temperature or temperature and relative humidity are high and (2) taking in plenty of fluids prior to and during exercise. Although quite popular, the practice of taking salt tablets for the prevention of heat stress is not recommended. Contrary to popular belief, the lack of salt is rarely the cause of heat stress, and taking salt tablets may simply contribute to dehydration and, therefore, to heat stress itself. When heat illness does occur, it may take one of three forms: (1) heat cramps, (2) heat exhaustion, or (3) heat stroke.

Heat Cramps

Heat cramps are simply muscle cramps caused by the forceful contraction of a muscle experiencing dehydration or a disturbance in its normal electrolyte balance. When muscle cramps occur during or following exercise, the cramp should be grasped firmly and held until it begins to relax. When the cramp has subsided, the calf (the most common site of heat-related muscle cramps) may be passively stretched. To reduce the risk of recurrence, fluids should be taken in.

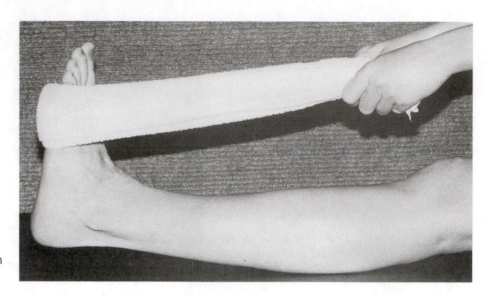

Once the cramp has subsided, gently stretch the muscle.

Heat Exhaustion

Heat exhaustion often occurs without the prior occurrence of heat cramps. Symptoms of heat exhaustion include nausea, dizziness, profuse sweating, and headache. With the onset of any of these or other related symptoms while walking in hot weather when heat illness might be suspected, you should discontinue exercise immediately and move to a cool area where you can lie down. You should use fanning or cool towels to lower body temperature and drink plenty of fluids. Heat exhaustion is potentially a very dangerous condition, since failure to recognize and care for it can result in its progression toward heat stroke.

Heat Stroke

Heat stroke represents the failure of the body's thermoregulatory (temperature-regulating) system. Should this occur, the results are potentially life-threatening. Therefore, recognition and prompt response are vital. While many of the symptoms of heat stroke are similar to those of heat exhaustion, only more advanced, this condition is characterized by extremely high body temperatures (over 104°), an absence of sweating, loss of muscle tone, and possibly seizure and/or coma. When heat stroke is suspected, the victim must be cooled rapidly using fanning, cold towels, cold water, and so forth, and transported immediately to a medical facility so that medical care can be provided.

Summary

Fitness walking is basically a safe, enjoyable, and beneficial activity. However, injury and, to a lesser degree, illness are occasionally encountered. Most exercise-related injury and illness problems can be prevented with a thorough understanding and utilization of sound exercise principles, selection of proper exercise equipment, proper use of warm-up and cool-down techniques, and knowing when exercise should be discontinued or not done at all. When unavoidable injury or illness does occur, proper self-care should be employed for mild injury and illness, while more serious conditions should be referred to a physician for evaluation and treatment.

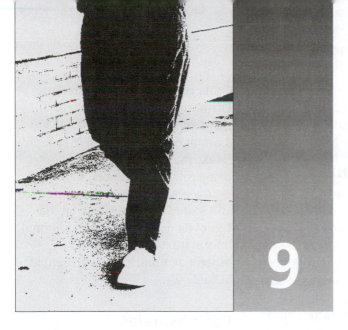

Nutrition

If there were one perfect substitute for the nutrients provided us in food, you can be sure that everyone would know about it.

Ronda Gates

9

"You are what you eat." This old and familiar adage implies that nutrition is the primary determining factor in our growth, development, and, ultimately, fitness and health. While this may be a bit of an overstatement, it is true that our diet does influence our health in a variety of ways. Unfortunately, however, many people have come to believe that nutrition holds the key to both our health problems and our quest for personal fitness. Each year, Americans spend billions of dollars on so called "health foods," nutrition supplements, and diet plans. Two major truths characterize the role that nutrition plays in the health and fitness of an individual: First, poor nutritional practices can, and often do, contribute to a decline in personal health and/or fitness. Second, special foods, supplements, or nutritional plans will do little, if anything, to enhance health and fitness beyond that which can be obtained through a basic, well-balanced diet.

Food = Nutrients

The foods we eat are made up of specialized components called *nutrients*, approximately 50 of which are necessary for a person to grow, develop, and function properly. Some nutrients are identified as *essential nutrients*, meaning that (1) they are necessary for the body to function, and (2) they cannot be manufactured by the body in sufficient quantities and must be taken in through the foods we eat (e.g., iron, vitamin C, protein).

Foods and the nutrients that they contain perform three basic functions in the body. First, some nutrients (primarily carbohydrates and fats) provide energy or fuel for the body. Second, nutrients such as protein and calcium function in building and maintaining body tissues. Finally, several nutrients help regulate body functions such as iodine (thyroid function) and vitamin K (blood clotting).

Nutrients may be classified in four groups: macronutrients,

micronutrients, water, and dietary fiber. Let's learn more about each in the following sections.

Macronutrients

Three nutrients—protein, carbohydrates, and fat—are known as *macronutrients,* because they are needed in relatively large quantities (*macro* means large) in our diet. While these three nutrients perform a variety of important functions, they all share one characteristic. Macronutrients are the only direct source of energy (calories) in the foods we eat. Therefore, they play an important role in exercise (energy) and weight management (calorie intake).

Protein

Among fitness enthusiasts and athletes, protein has long been afforded a special place of honor in the diet, due to the common misconception that protein is the source of big, strong muscles. Proteins are simply specialized compounds made up of chemicals called *amino acids*. They may be obtained from a wide variety of foods, although the protein found in animal foods (meat, fish, poultry, dairy products, etc.) is of higher quality than that found in plant foods, since animal protein generally contains all the essential amino acids.

Proteins play several roles in the body, from maintaining healthy hair and nails to regulating the oxygen-carrying efficiency of the blood. And, while it is true that muscle is composed of a significant amount of protein, muscle size and strength are basically functions of genetic endowment, body hormones, and strength development exercise. Contrary to popular belief, no scientific evidence indicates that the intake of extra protein or amino acids will enhance muscle size or strength. Furthermore, because protein metabolism requires a significant amount of water, excessive protein intake may produce potentially dangerous dehydration. Finally, excess protein may be converted to and stored as fat, a situation that few of us need or desire. Additional information on protein and the other macronutrients is presented in Table 9.1.

Carbohydrates

Carbohydrates are sugars (simple carbohydrates) and starches (complex carbohydrates). Because of their ease of digestion and utilization (Figure 9.1), carbohydrates provide the body with its most convenient source of energy. Carbohydrates are found throughout the diet in foods easily recognized as sweets and starchy foods. Refined table sugar is almost pure carbohydrate, but it contains virtually no other nutrients and thus is not highly recommended as a primary carbohydrate source. Fresh fruit, starchy vegetables, and pasta, however, are rich sources of carbohydrate, in addition to providing a vast array of other desirable nutrients such as protein, unsaturated fat, vitamins, minerals, water, and dietary fiber. Fitness enthusiasts and athletes have long recognized carbohydrates as a rich and efficient source of energy, and, as such, often consume carbohydrate-rich foods in an attempt to enhance energy production during exercise.

Although it is recommended that more than half of all calories eaten should be in carbohydrate form (see Table 9.1), a balanced diet will provide enough carbohydrates to meet the energy needs of most exercising adults. Also, as with protein and fat, the body will convert excess carbohydrates into body fat.

TABLE 9.1
Macronutrient Digestion

	Proteins	Carbohydrates	Fats
What are they?	Amino acid compounds	Sugars and starches	Fatty acid and glycerol compounds
Types?	Complete (animal) Incomplete (plant)	Simple (sugars) Complex (starches)	Saturated, Unsaturated
Where do we find them?	Variety of animal and plant sources	Sweets and starches	Variety of animal and plant sources
What do they do?	Tissue structure, numerous specific functions	Energy, numerous specific functions	Energy stores, cell integrity (e.g., skin), fat-soluble vitamins
How much do we need?	Approximately 1 gram per kilogram of body weight per day	No RDA	No RDA
Can we get too much?	YES—excess fat; dehydration	YES—excess fat	YES—excess fat; CHD risk
Recommended intake pattern?	Should emphasize complete	Should emphasize complex	Should emphasize unsaturated
Recommended Calorie intake?	10%–15%	55%–60%	25%–30%

Fat

Fat is the most calorie-rich of the macronutrients, with each gram containing 9 calories as opposed to 4 calories per gram with protein and carbohydrates. Dietary fat may be divided into two distinct categories: saturated and unsaturated. Saturated fat is generally found in animal foods (meat, dairy products, etc.), although some plant foods such as palm oil and coconut oil also contain saturated fat. Because of its known relationship to the development of cardiovascular disease, the intake of saturated fat should be limited. Unsaturated fat is most often found in plant oils such as corn and sunflower oils, and it is the preferred form of dietary fat, since there is no known direct link between unsaturated fat and cardiovascular disease.

In addition to being a rich source of energy (especially at rest and during aerobic exercise such as walking), fat is necessary for the development and maintenance of healthy skin as well as the transportation, absorption, and storage of fat-soluble vitamins A, D, E, and K. Research indicates that most Americans take in excessive amounts of fat, which, in part, contributes to the high rate of obesity and cardiovascular disease in our country.

Recommended Macronutrient Intake

How much protein, carbohydrate, and fat should one consume to meet the body's daily needs, maintain optimal weight and health, and support the energy demands of a regular exercise program? The answer to this question is not simple, but some basic guidelines should be considered. Since macronutrients

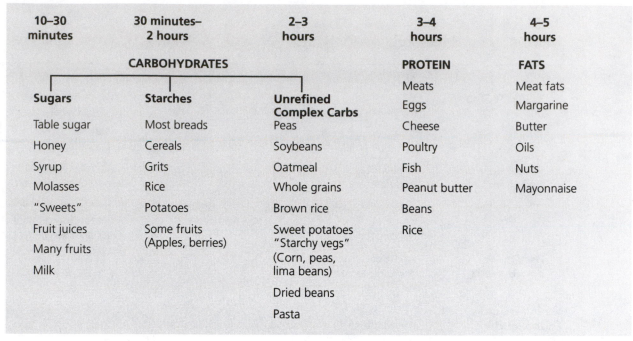

10–30 minutes	30 minutes–2 hours	2–3 hours	3–4 hours	4–5 hours
CARBOHYDRATES			**PROTEIN**	**FATS**
			Meats	Meat fats
Sugars	**Starches**	**Unrefined Complex Carbs**	Eggs	Margarine
Table sugar	Most breads	Peas	Cheese	Butter
Honey	Cereals	Soybeans	Poultry	Oils
Syrup	Grits	Oatmeal	Fish	Nuts
Molasses	Rice	Whole grains	Peanut butter	Mayonnaise
"Sweets"	Potatoes	Brown rice	Beans	
Fruit juices	Some fruits (Apples, berries)	Sweet potatoes "Starchy vegs" (Corn, peas, lima beans)	Rice	
Many fruits				
Milk		Dried beans		
		Pasta		

Figure 9.1 Macronutrient Digestion

are the only source of calorie intake, you must first be sure that you are taking in enough protein, carbohydrates, and fat (and thus calories) to meet your daily energy needs. This may be determined by comparing your daily calorie intake with your daily energy expenditure, a procedure discussed in detail in Chapter 10.

There is no fixed recommendation for the daily intake of carbohydrates or fats. It is, however, recommended that adults take in approximately 1 gram of protein per kilogram of body weight each day. To determine how much protein you should take in on a daily basis, simply divide your body weight (in pounds) by 2.2 to convert to kilograms, and this will be the approximate number of grams of protein that your daily diet should contain. Because of the wide variety of protein sources available in the typical American diet, few people fail to meet this daily protein intake recommendation.

It is also important that you attempt to get your daily calories from a balance of the three macronutrients. As stated previously, each gram of protein and carbohydrate contains 4 calories, while a gram of fat contains 9 calories. Most (55% to 60%) of one's caloric intake should be in the form of carbohydrates, with the emphasis placed on eating complex (starches) rather than simple (sugar) carbohydrates. Fat should comprise no more that 30% (preferably 25% or less) of calories (unsaturated fats should be emphasized), while the balance (10% to 15%) should be in the form of protein. For example, for a 2,000-calorie per day diet, 1,100 to 1,200 calories should be from carbohydrates, 500 to 600 from fat, and 200 to 300 from protein.

Micronutrients

Vitamins and minerals are among the most familiar of all nutrients.

They are often referred to as *micro-nutrients,* since they are needed in very small amounts.

Vitamins

Vitamins are organic compounds that are essential to the normal functioning of the body. There are 13 known vitamins, most of which must be taken in regularly through the food we eat. Each vitamin performs a variety of specific and unique roles in the normal functioning of the body, a detailed discussion of which is beyond the scope of this book. Many function as enzymes or coenzymes, which simply means that they help regulate the efficiency of such important bodily functions as the manufacture of healthy blood cells and the conversion of carbohydrates and fat to energy.

Vitamins are of two basic types: fat-soluble and water-soluble. Fat-soluble vitamins (A, D, E, and K) are transported, absorbed, and stored along with body fat. For this reason, they are not easily eliminated by the body and may be stored in rather large amounts. If excessive amounts of fat-soluble vitamins are consumed (as with megadoses of vitamin supplements), they may produce toxic, health-threatening effects. Therefore, contrary to popular belief, taking in large amounts of vitamins may not merely be unnecessary but may be potentially dangerous.

Minerals

Nutrient minerals are inorganic compounds that are essential to the normal functioning of the body. Of the 20 known minerals, most must be consumed on a regular basis, and are found in a vast variety of foods. Just as with vitamins, minerals perform very specific functions in the body, from tissue building and repair (e.g., calcium promotes healthy bones and teeth) to regulating metabolism (e.g., iodine regulates thyroid function) and other vital bodily functions (e.g., iron contributes to oxygen delivery in the blood).

Six minerals (calcium, phosphorous, magnesium, potassium, sodium, and chloride) are called *major minerals* because they are needed in amounts greater than 100 milligrams/day, while the balance of the minerals (iron, zinc, iodine, etc.) are needed in smaller amounts, thus classified as *trace minerals*. The excessive intake of some minerals (usually occurring only when supplements are taken) may be potentially dangerous to one's health. For recommended intake information concerning both vitamins and minerals, consult a standard RDA (Recommended Dietary Allowance) chart.

Other Essential Nutrients

In addition to protein, carbohydrates, fats, vitamins, and minerals, two other nutrients are essential to normal body functioning and optimal health: water and dietary fiber.

Water

Water is perhaps the most important yet most often overlooked of the essential nutrients. Water is essential for a variety of important body processes, including (1) digestion (hydrolysis), (2) the transportation of nutrients and waste products (blood circulation and urination), (3) the maintenance of normal tissue consistency (blood), and (4) temperature regulation (perspiration/evaporation).

Under normal conditions, an adult will lose approximately 2 to 2.5 liters of water every day, through perspiration, urination, respiration, and body metabolism. Other circumstances such as hot weather and exercise will cause additional water loss. Therefore, a person needs to consume water throughout the day and should increase water consumption when exposed to a hot environment and/or exercising. Fortunately, in addition to existing in its common beverage form, water is found throughout the diet in beverages such as milk, tea, and juices and in fresh fruits and vegetables.

Dietary Fiber

Dietary fiber is basically a nondigestible form of plant carbohydrate. Since humans do not possess the enzymes necessary for its digestion, fiber passes through the digestive tract without being absorbed as other nutrients are. The value of fiber in the diet has been actively researched in recent years, and it has been determined that fiber promotes the normal movement and elimination of solid wastes from the body. Medical research indicates that failure of the body's solid waste elimination system to perform properly may place a person at increased risk of developing colon and/or rectal cancer. Therefore, it is recommended that foods rich in fiber (raw fruits and vegetables, whole-grain products, etc.) be included in the daily diet.

Nutrition and Health

Proper nutrition has long been considered an important component of a healthy lifestyle. In recognition of the relationship between nutrition and health, the U.S. Departments of Agriculture and Health and Human Services have published the following *Dietary Guidelines for Americans* (Figure 9.2).

Aim for Fitness

When it comes to a healthy lifestyle, good nutrition and regular physical activity go hand in hand. Therefore, although not literally "dietary" in nature, the first two recommendations address the importance of maintaining a healthy weight and engaging in daily physical activity.

Aim for a Healthy Weight

Proper nutrition is essential to maintaining a healthy body weight. Excess body fat has been linked to such health problems as cardiovascular disease, diabetes, stress on weight-supporting bones and joints, and the inability to regulate body temperature in hot weather. A detailed discussion of weight management is presented in Chapter 10.

Be Physically Active Each Day

Daily physical activity has long been recognized as one of the major components of a healthy lifestyle. As noted in Chapter 4, vigorous aerobic exercise such as fitness walking should be done 4 to 5 days a week to improve aerobic fitness. However, every day should include some form of physical activity if one is to truly live an active lifestyle. In keeping with the saying that variety is the spice of life, enjoy other activities in addition to your fitness walking to create a well-rounded active lifestyle.

Build a Healthy Base

Positive nutrition must be based on healthy food choices. Using the USDA Food Pyramid, eating a variety of healthy foods and practicing food safety are important in "building a healthy base."

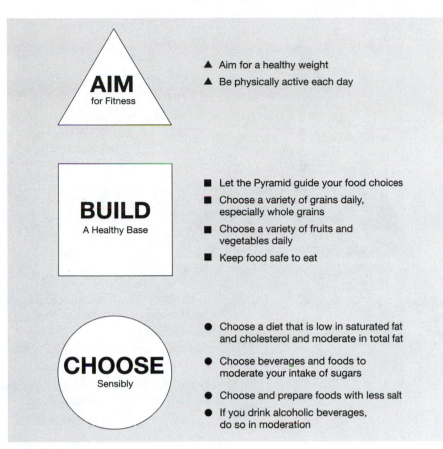

Figure 9.2 2000 Dietary Guidelines for Americans

Furthermore, as discussed earlier, plant foods are truly cholesterol-free. Therefore, it is recommended that the daily diet contain a variety of grain products.

Choose a Variety of Fruits and Vegetables Daily

This recommendation is based on the same nutritional benefits identified earlier for grains. Fruits and vegetables are high in complex carbohydrates, vitamins, minerals, and fiber, while containing little (if any) fat and no cholesterol.

Keep Food Safe to Eat

In recent years, concerns about food safety have become a major health issue. Food that is improperly prepared (e.g., unwashed fruits and vegetables), cooked (e.g., undercooked meat), and/or stored (e.g., leaving cooked food out of the refrigerator, resulting in spoilage) has been linked to a wide variety of food-borne diseases, some of which may even result in death. Therefore, it is imperative that food be cleaned, prepared, and stored according to established methods of safe food handling.

Choose Sensibly

Sensible food choices will go a long way toward establishing a healthy nutritional lifestyle. Moderation is the key to recommendations concerning the consumption of fat, sugar, salt, and alcohol.

Choose a Diet Low in Saturated Fat and Cholesterol and Moderate in Total Fat

Research indicates that the typical American diet contains entirely too much fat. Excessive dietary fat, especially saturated fat, has been shown to increase one's risk of

Let the Pyramid Guide Your Food Choices

Among the most recent attempts to provide Americans with a sound, easy-to-understand plan for healthy eating is the USDA Food Pyramid (Figure 9.3). Using the Pyramid as your guide to food choices is an excellent way to build variety into your daily diet.

Choose a Variety of Grains Daily, Especially Whole Grains

Grain products (breads, cereals, pasta, etc.) contain a wide variety of vitamins and minerals, as well as being a rich source of complex carbohydrates and dietary fiber. As with all plant foods, grains are generally low in fat, therefore offering the double benefit of quality nutrition without adding to dietary fat intake.

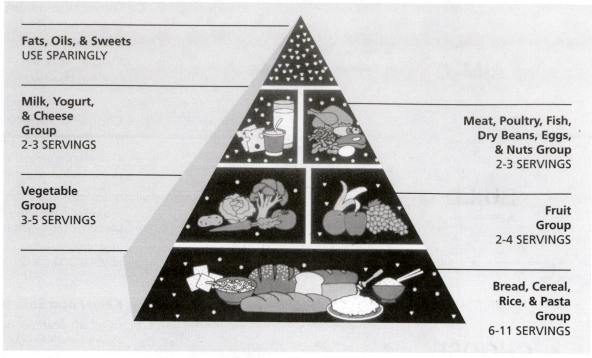

Figure 9.3 Food Pyramid

obesity and certain types of cancer (e.g., breast and colon/rectal) and, along with dietary cholesterol, is believed to contribute directly to cardiovascular disease, the number one killer in the United States today.

As stated earlier, fat is a necessary component of a healthy diet. However, total dietary fat should be limited to no more than 30% of calorie intake, with no more than one-third of this amount coming in the form of saturated fats (animal fats and tropical plant oils). Furthermore, dietary cholesterol should be reduced to a minimum, by limiting the amount of animal products (meat, shellfish, dairy products, etc.) consumed on a daily basis, since cholesterol is found only in animal foods. Some practical suggestions for lowering fat and cholesterol in the diet include substituting low-fat milk for whole milk, trimming visible fat from meats before cooking, removing skin from chicken before eating, cooking with unsaturated oils, baking and broiling rather than frying, substituting low-fat yogurt or sherbet for ice cream and angel food cake for regular cake, and occasionally eating meatless meals.

Choose Beverages and Foods to Moderate Your Intake of Sugars

Sugars are a popular part of the American diet. Though a rich source of carbohydrates, the calories gained from sugars are often called "empty" or "diluted" calories, meaning that the calories are accompanied by few, if any, additional nutrients, thus weakening their broad nutritional value. On the other hand, a baked potato offers not only a rich source of calories but a variety of vitamins and minerals, as well as dietary fiber. Also, high-sugar snack foods often contain a significant amount of fat. The excessive intake of sugar and sugar-rich foods may contribute to obesity as well as an increased likelihood of dental cavities. Therefore, sugars should be consumed in moderate amounts by limiting sugar-rich snacks, substituting fruits for processed sugar snack foods, and reducing the amount of table sugar added to foods and beverages.

Choose and Prepare Foods with Less Salt

Health experts agree that Americans eat too much salt. One of the major components of salt is sodium. In some people, excessive sodium intake may contribute to the development of high blood pressure, a potentially serious health problem. While not everyone appears to experience this sensitivity to sodium, even those without high blood pressure may reduce their risk of getting it by controlling the amount of salt in the diet.

At the present time, no accurate way is available to predict who may develop high blood pressure, but it is recommended that limiting salt intake is a prudent practice for most people. Suggestions for limiting dietary salt include using non-sodium seasonings such as herbs and lemon juice instead of salt; eating more fresh vegetables rather than canned ones; selecting fresh rather than canned or processed meat, fish, and poultry; and substituting low-salt snacks for highly salted chips, crackers, and nuts.

If You Drink Alcoholic Beverages, Do So in Moderation

Nutritionally, alcoholic beverages have little to offer other than empty calories. Beverage alcohol has a high caloric value (1 gram = 7 calories) but few, if any, nutrients. Also, alcohol is the most commonly abused drug in the United States,

accounting for numerous injuries, deaths, and other social problems each year.

Alcohol abuse may contribute to cardiovascular disease, various forms of cancer, and potentially fatal liver disease. In addition, alcohol is a powerful diuretic, which simulates the production and release of urine from the body. When accompanied by hot weather and/or exercise, the excessive loss of body fluids may lead to dehydration, heat illness, and possibly death. The best advice is, if you choose to drink alcohol, do so in moderation.

Nutrition and Fitness

Historically, people have looked to nutrition for help in improving physical fitness and athletic performance. From secret herbs to powdered lions' teeth; exercisers have eaten, drunk, and taken a vast array of foods, beverages, and nutrition supplements in an attempt to become stronger, run faster and longer, and jump higher.

To what extent can nutrition enhance fitness? As stated in the opening part of this chapter, poor nutrition may reduce our capacity for optimal fitness. However, this does not mean that fitness can be improved through special diets, nutrition supplements, and other popular practices. To explore the truth about nutrition and fitness, let's take a look at some commonly asked questions.

As a Fitness Walker, Are My Nutritional Needs Different From Someone Who Does Not Exercise?

Not really. While it is true that exercise may increase your need for calories (see Chapter 10), even the most avid exerciser or athlete in heavy training can meet this need by adding calories to the daily diet. Since carbohydrates are the most easily digested and utilized source of calories, anyone engaged in regular aerobic exercise such as walking may consider increasing both the amount and percentage (55% to 60%, up to 65% to 70%) of carbohydrate calories in the daily diet. However, unless you are involved in heavy aerobic training (e.g., training for competitive distance racing), taking in extra calories will do little more than increase your chances of gaining unwanted fat. In short, most, if not all of the nutritional needs of a fitness walker may be easily met through a good, balanced diet.

Are Complex Carbohydrates Better for Me Than Sugar?

Yes. As pointed out earlier, complex carbohydrates (starches) are generally better for you than sugars for several reasons. In addition to being a rich source of carbohydrates, they usually contain other nutrients such as vitamins, minerals, and dietary fiber. Of perhaps greater interest to the fitness walker, complex carbohydrates are digested and absorbed somewhat more slowly than sugars. This "time-released" action results in less dramatic fluctuations in blood sugar levels, providing a more steady conversion of dietary carbohydrate into energy.

Will Taking in Extra Protein Enhance My Fitness?

No. Big, strong muscles do not come from protein-rich foods or protein supplements but from genetic endowment, hormone influence, and heavy resistance exercise (strength training). Furthermore, protein has little direct influence on aerobic fitness. In view of these facts, along with the potential dangers of excessive protein intake (cellular dehydration, unwanted fat gain, etc.), the intake of extra protein is neither necessary for optimal fitness nor recommended.

Can I Meet My Nutritional Needs with a Vegetarian Diet?

Yes. A true vegetarian diet consists of only plant foods. It is less likely to be high in fat, saturated fat, and cholesterol and will very likely contain most of the essential vitamins and minerals and a significant amount of dietary fiber. Therefore, with careful planning, a vegetarian diet may supply virtually all the nutrients found in a meat-based diet, with the added advantages of fewer calories, less fat, and no cholesterol.

A couple of cautions should be noted, however. First, plant foods do not contain the essential vitamin, B_{12}. Therefore, the true vegetarian should consult his or her physician concerning other sources of the vitamin. Second, the protein found in plant foods is generally missing one or more of the essential amino acids, so eating a wide variety of protein-rich vegetables is necessary if one is to get all the necessary amino acids.

Should I Eat Extra Salt or Take Salt Tablets When Exercising?

No. Most Americans get more than enough salt in their diet, and that includes those who exercise regularly. Exercise-related heat problems (See chapter 8) have long been thought to be related to the loss of salt through perspiration. However, sodium (salt) loss rarely is the cause of heat illness. On the contrary, excessive salt, especially in concentrated form such as salt tablets, may actually contribute to dehydration and may be a contributing factor in the development of heat illness. The intake of extra salt before or during exercise (even in hot weather) not only is ineffective but may be potentially dangerous.

What Is the Best Replacement Fluid When I Am Exercising?

For moderate to vigorous exercise such as fitness walking, the best replacement beverage is usually water. The primary purpose of fluids consumed before, during, and after exercise is to prevent dehydration, which can inhibit performance and pose a danger to your health.

A host of sports drinks have been developed and marketed on the premise that they are superior to water for fluid replacement because they contain other important additives. Most of these drinks contain some combination of specialized minerals called electrolytes (sodium, potassium, and chloride), since these are lost in small amounts when you perspire. Many also contain glucose polymers (complex carbohydrates) in an attempt to provide the consumer with additional energy for exercise. Most of these specialty beverages contain some form of sugar and flavoring to make the drink taste good. The use of specialized sports drinks remains controversial, at best. However, most experts agree that, for moderate to vigorous exercise, water is the best fluid for combating exercise-related dehydration.

Will Nutritional Supplements Enhance My Fitness?

No. Contrary to popular belief, no scientific evidence supports the belief that supplements such as vitamins, minerals, wheat germ, bee pollen, or amino acids will improve fitness. The best nutritional path to fitness is a balanced diet.

Does It Really Matter What I Eat before I Exercise?

Not really. The food you eat prior to a walk or other form of exercise will require several hours to digest completely and be available for your body to use (see Figure 9.1). Therefore, it will have little if any direct effect on your ability to exercise, unless, of course, you eat something that doesn't agree with you. If you plan to eat before walking, choose foods that are not likely to cause gastric upset while exercising, and allow at least 30 minutes between the meal and the beginning of your walk.

Are All Snacks Unhealthy?

No. Smaller, more frequent meals may actually be more beneficial to the body than the commonly accepted three-meals-a-day plan. Eating between meals can, and often is, a desirable alternative to three large meals. The essential element to consider, however, is what kinds of foods make up these between meal snacks. Empty-calorie foods that provide little or no nutritional value other than calories should be avoided or at least limited. Examples of such high-fat and/or high-calorie foods are doughnuts, ice cream, candy, and potato chips. The following list

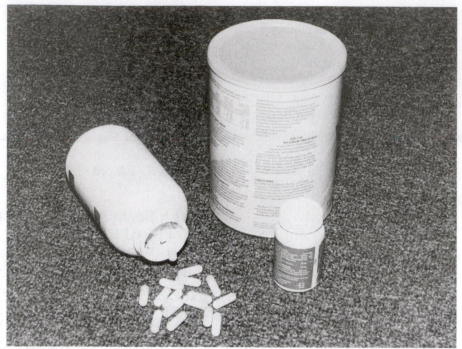

Bee pollen, vitamins, protein powder, and other diet supplements are no substitute for good nutrition.

- Baked chips—a reduced fat alternative to regular snack chips.
- Sherbet—great low-fat substitute for ice cream.
- Soft drinks—most contain sugar and little else and therefore should be used in moderation. Sugar-free (aspartame-sweetened) beverage products may be a suitable alternative.

Research indicates that the average daily American diet is made up of 15% to 20% snack calories. When that sinking feeling indicates that the "fuel tank" is on low, it would be a good idea to have nutritious snacks available. Moderation is the key to sensible snacking. Place the amount you plan to eat in a dish, and put the rest away. Avoid eating straight out of the bag or package, and develop the habit of stopping when the dish is empty.

contains snack foods that are not only tasty but nutritious as well:

- Fresh fruits—high in complex carbohydrates, vitamins, minerals, and fiber, and virtually fat-free.
- Fresh vegetables—high in complex carbohydrates (low-fat dip is optional), vitamins, minerals, and fiber, and virtually fat-free.
- Cereals—many contain no fat and relatively low sugar content while providing complex carbohydrates and fiber.
- Popcorn—preferably air popped, "light" oil varieties; good source of fiber.
- Yogurt—nonfat and low-fat varieties are often as tasty as fat-full flavors.
- Popsicles—may contain sugar but are fat-free.
- Angel food cake—contains few nutrients but is fat-free.
- Cookies—Fig Newtons and ginger snaps are among the lowest in fat content.

Summary

An important part of any fitness program is proper nutrition. A good diet provides your body with the necessary materials for building and maintaining body tissues, regulating body functions, and producing the energy necessary to meet your daily energy needs. There is no substitute for a well-balanced diet that contains the recommended amounts of carbohydrate, protein, fat, vitamins, minerals, water, and dietary fiber. Special diets and nutritional gimmicks will not enhance fitness or improve athletic performance. However, by understanding the various roles that nutrients play in your body and following accepted dietary guidelines, you can establish nutritional habits that can help you stay healthy throughout your life.

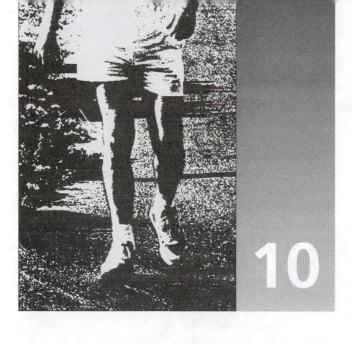

10

*Become aerobically fit, and fat
(and weight) will take care of itself.*
Covert Bailey

Weight Management

Few health-related subjects receive as much media attention
as weight control. Nearly one of
every three Americans weighs more
than they should, posing a direct
threat to both their health and their
enjoyment of life. Thin is in, and
some 20 million Americans diet on
a regular basis, including about
one-half the adult female population. Unfortunately, dieting alone
has never proven very successful for
effective weight reduction, mainly
because dieting offers only a temporary solution to a permanent
problem. Weight management is a
complex issue that simply cannot
be resolved through dieting.

Body Composition

How much you weigh is not as important as the specific makeup of
your body weight. When considering
body weight, the human body can
be described as having two general
types of tissue: fat and fat-free
(bone, muscle, water, etc.). The
relative amount of fat and fat-free
weight is known as *body composition* (Figure 10.1).

Fat Weight

Fat is a necessary part of a healthy
body. Not only does fat represent
the body's richest source of stored
energy; it also insulates and protects
vital organs, contributes to efficient
neurological function, is an important structural component of cell
membranes, and is necessary for
the utilization of fat-soluble vitamins. Body fat may be divided into
two categories: essential fat and
expendable fat. *Essential fat* is that
portion of the body's fat that is necessary for the maintenance of good
health. In men, essential fat makes
up about 2% to 4% of the total body
weight, whereas in females, essential fat constitutes about 10% to
12% of total weight. *Expendable fat*

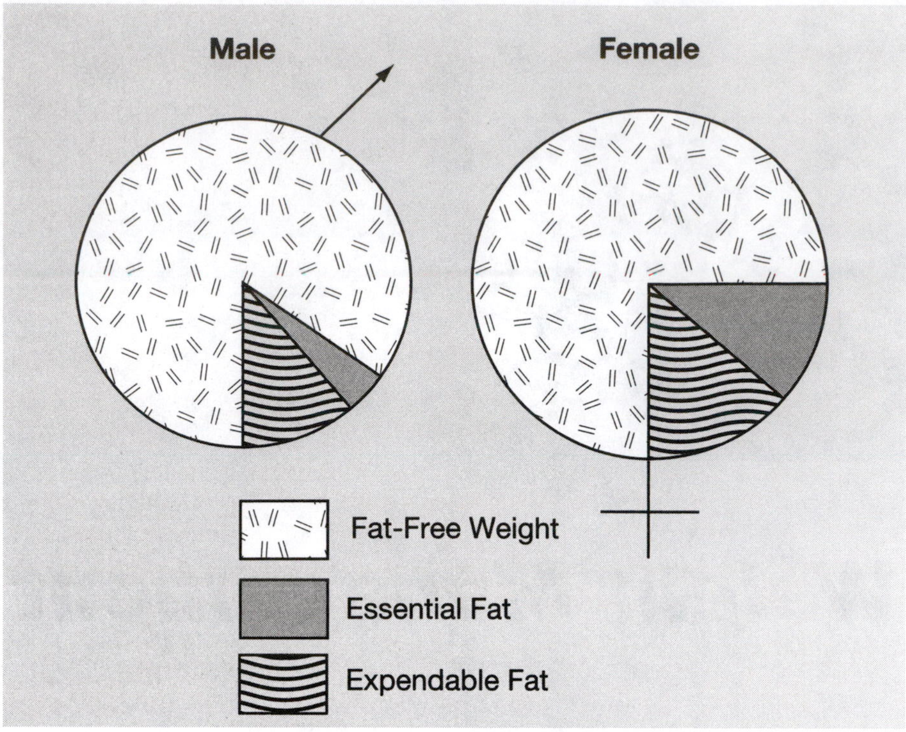

Figure 10.1 Typical Body Composition

is that portion of the body's stored fat that is in excess of the essential fat. It is the body's expendable stored fat that may be reduced during effective weight loss.

Fat-Free Weight

The body's fat-free weight is made up of all tissue other than fat—muscle, bone, and body fluids. Unlike fat, many fat-free tissues (especially muscle) are metabolically active, meaning that they must have energy to support their activities. Therefore, the more active fat-free tissue becomes (as with exercise), the more energy (calories) that tissue "burns." This concept is critical to understanding the dynamics of weight loss and maintenance that will be discussed later.

Overweight or Overfat?

When a person weighs more than is considered desirable, he or she is often referred to as overweight. Traditionally, height-weight charts have been used to determine the optimal weight for persons of various heights and body frame sizes. While this process is simple and easily understood, it is not considered highly reliable. Equating body weight with health risk implies that you may step on the scale, read your weight, and accurately determine whether your current weight is appropriate for your body. In other words, two people who are the same sex, height, and weight, should possess about equal weight-related health risks. However, it is quite possible that one may be quite lean, having relatively little body fat, while the other may have a substantial amount of excess body fat. Body weight, therefore, is not always a

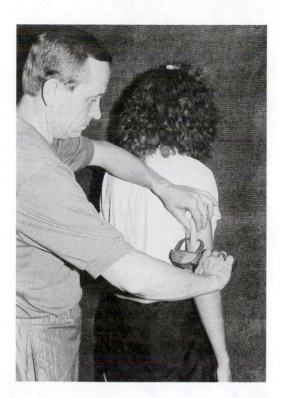

Skinfold measurement is an easy and accurate way to assess body composition.

good indicator of body composition. "Overfat" may be a more accurate way to describe a person who has excessive body fat that, if not reduced, may pose a serious health threat.

What, then, constitutes excessive body fat? Most experts agree that an adult male should have no more than 12% to 18% body fat, while an adult female should not exceed 18% to 24% body fat. Therefore, anyone who exceeds these recommended standards would be considered overfat, while a person who is 20% or more above the recommended standard would be classified as obese.

Currently, the most accurate way to measure body composition is through a laboratory procedure known as *hydrostatic* (underwater) *weighing*. This process requires that the body be weighed twice: once out of the water and once while totally submerged underwater. Since fat is less dense than muscle, it tends to float. Therefore, by applying some

rather complex statistical procedures, one's dry and underwater weights may be used to assess body composition accurately.

Since hydrostatic weighing is time-consuming and requires specialized equipment, a variety of simpler methods have been developed, the most popular of which is skinfold measurement. Since much of the body's stored fat may be found just below the surface of the skin, the thickness of fat deposits at specific sites may be used to estimate body composition. Although considered less accurate than underwater weighing, skinfold measurement is widely accepted as a reasonable alternative for predicting body fat percentages.

Numerous "high-tech" methods for assessing body composition are currently under investigation, but, to date, none have been determined to offer the accuracy or reliability of underwater weighing and skinfold measurement.

Health Risks of Overfatness

Research indicates that excessive body fat may be related to a host of potentially serious health problems. Among the most common are cardiovascular disease, orthopedic (bone and joint) stress, thermoregulatory (body temperature) problems, diabetes, and an increased probability of living a sedentary (inactive) lifestyle.

Cardiovascular Disease

As stated earlier, body fat is basically inactive. Therefore, unlike muscle, it provides additional body weight without contributing to the work output of the body. In a real sense, excessive body fat may be viewed as parasitic, in that it requires blood flow and nourishment, while offering little in return. As body fat increases, so does the tendency to develop several forms of cardiovascular disease, including coronary artery disease and hypertension (chronic high blood pressure).

Orthopedic Stress

Excess body fat adds excess weight to the body. This weight must be supported by the feet, ankles, legs, knees, hips, and lower back. Over time, the stress on these supportive structures caused by excess fat may contribute to annoying pain, discomfort, and eventually degenerative (arthritic-like) joint injury.

Thermoregulatory Problems

When the body becomes hot (because of hot weather, exercising, etc.), it dissipates heat via the evaporation of perspiration from the skin. This process is necessary for the body to avoid overheating, resulting in heat exhaustion or heat stroke. Fat is a very efficient insulator, and as such, it helps the body retain heat during cold weather exposure. However, in hot weather or when exercising, excessive fat will inhibit the body's ability to cool, thus predisposing the person to potentially serious heat illness.

Diabetes

Diabetes is characterized by the body's inability to manufacture insulin of sufficient quality or quantity to facilitate the absorption of sugar into body cells. Excess body fat has been shown to increase the body's need for insulin and therefore may directly contribute to the onset of some types of diabetes.

Sedentary Lifestyle

The more excess fat a person has, the more difficulty he or she is likely to have participating in and enjoying physical activity. Not only does this sedentary lifestyle deprive the person of the many health benefits and enjoyment of regular exercise, but it also may contribute directly to the accumulation of additional body fat, thus increasing the likelihood of health problems.

Others

In addition to the specific health problems already identified, research continues to uncover information linking excess body fat with other health-threatening conditions. The person with excess body fat may be *more susceptible to infectious disease* and will tend to *heal less quickly following an injury or surgery.* Overfatness and obesity have been associated with an *increased frequency of accident-related injury.* One's risk of *certain types of cancers* may be increased with excess body fat. Moreover, although often overlooked when considering the potential health risks of overfatness and obesity, numerous *psychological and emotional problems* may be at least partially the result of one being overfat in our "thin is in" culture.

Metabolism— A Key Concept

No concept is more critical to understanding the dynamics of weight gain and weight loss than that of the body's metabolism. *Metabolism* is the sum total of all the body's chemical and physical processes, plus the energy (calories) expended in carrying out those processes. Simply stated, the higher your metabolism, the more calories your body burns, and the less likely you are to accumulate excess fat.

Some people are called "slow gainers" because they seem to be able to eat virtually anything without gaining a pound, while others are often referred to as "fast gainers" because they appear to gain weight just by looking at food. The secret to this unfair situation may simply be that the slow gainer's metabolism is higher, thus making that person more resistant to unwanted weight gain.

The key, then, is to identify those things that decrease and increase metabolic rate and use them to your advantage to attain and maintain your desired weight. Four factors that lower metabolism, and therefore, make you susceptible to unwanted weight gain, are (1) age, (2) fasting, (3) loss of lean body tissue (muscle), and (4) inactivity.

As the body ages, your metabolism will tend to slow down. The slowing of metabolic rate usually begins at about age 30, and it decreases at a rate of about 2% for each decade thereafter. Therefore,

you can expect your metabolism to decline by about 2% when in your 30s, another 2% during your 40s, and so on. This is one reason that many adults begin to gain weight when they pass 30, even though they may not be eating more or exercising less.

Dieting in an attempt to lose weight will produce only short-term, temporary weight loss, since the body will respond to a cutback in food intake by slowing the metabolism. This is basically a protective mechanism designed to protect the body against starvation during periods of fasting. For the dieter, however, this fasting response can prove very frustrating, because, the less he or she eats, the more the body's metabolism slows, making further weight loss even more difficult.

Another negative effect of extreme dieting without exercise is the loss of lean body tissue (muscle). Since muscle tissue is metabolically active, any loss of muscle will lower the body's metabolism and thus its demand for energy (calories).

Finally, a sedentary lifestyle will result in a lower metabolism, because inactivity often results in the loss of metabolically active muscle tissue and a gain in inactive body fat. As the metabolism slows, you will find that physical activity becomes more difficult, causing you to become even more inactive—and the vicious cycle continues.

Therefore, to attain and maintain a desirable body weight, you should consider the following tips:

1. Be aware of the natural decline in metabolic rate that accompanies the aging process.

2. Avoid severe calorie restriction diets.

3. Do not diet without exercising regularly, too, to preserve lean muscle.

4. Resist the temptation to become a member of the local chapter of "Couch Potatoes Anonymous."

Weight Gain/Loss Concepts

Several theories have been proposed to explain why people gain and lose weight. Research indicates that at least four such theories have scientific merit, and these may help explain the weight gain/weight loss process.

Energy Balance Concept

The oldest and most familiar of the weight loss theories is the energy balance concept. Simply stated, the energy balance concept is based on the notion that if your daily energy intake (food) equals your daily energy expenditure (metabolism), your body weight will remain steady. Therefore, if your energy intake exceeds your energy expenditure, the result will be weight gain; and if your energy expenditure exceeds your energy intake, you will lose weight (Figure 10.2).

Research has shown that an imbalance between calories (energy) consumed and expended can result in weight gain and weight loss. However, anyone who has tried to lose weight through simply reducing calories has discovered that the initial rate of weight loss soon begins to slow and may even plateau, even though the lower-calorie diet is still being consumed. As described earlier, this reaction is the body's natural response to decreased food intake, and it will necessitate the use of exercise to offset this normal decline in metabolism.

To make practical use of the energy balance concept, you must have two pieces of information: your daily caloric intake and your daily energy expenditure. Your daily caloric intake can be easily estimated by carefully listing all of the foods eaten and then using a calorie table (found in any nutrition book) to compute the total number of calories consumed.

To estimate your daily caloric expenditure, you must first calculate your estimated basal metabolic rate (BMR), the amount of energy required to sustain the body's life support systems (see Figures 10.3 and 10.4 and Appendix D). Once BMR has been adjusted for age and body build, the next step is the calculation of preexercise metabolic rate (PXMR). Preexercise metabolic rate includes the amount of energy used for the digestion, absorption, and utilization of food (often referred to as the *thermic effect* of food, or TEF) and for the completion of light daily activity. It may be estimated by adding 20% to one's adjusted BMR. The final step in calculating one's estimated total daily energy expenditure involves adding the amount of energy expended through daily exercise (Tables 10.1 and 10.2) to the PXMR. This will provide you with your estimated total metabolic rate (TMR) or total daily energy expenditure. Simply stated, your total daily energy expenditure (TMR) = your BMR + 20% (estimate for TEF and light activity) + calories burned through exercise.

By comparing your total daily caloric intake with your total estimated energy expenditure (TMR), it is easy to determine whether you are likely to experience weight gain or weight loss and to adjust accordingly. Since 1 pound of body fat equals 3,500 calories, adjusting

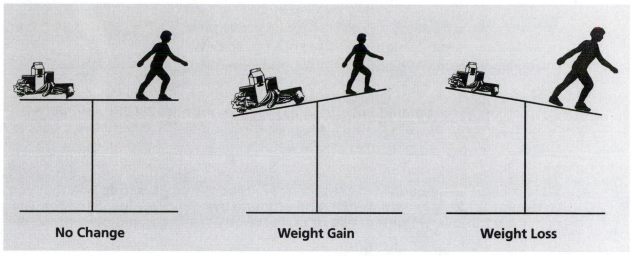

Figure 10.2 Energy Balance Concept

your calorie intake and exercise expenditure to produce a daily calorie deficit of 500 calories should result in weight loss of approximately 1 pound per week. However, energy balance is not the only factor that determines the rate of weight loss and gain.

Set Point Concept

Although the exact process is unknown, it is believed that each person has a weight-regulating mechanism (possibly in the hypothalamus of the brain) that assists the body in maintaining a certain body weight. This "preferred" body weight is often referred to as your *set point,* since it is relatively easily maintained and not easily changed. Each person's set point appears to be highly personal and rarely coincides with the most desirable weight for optimal health and well-being.

When you attempt to lose weight, thus moving below the body's established set point, your body will attempt to compensate for the weight loss by slowing its metabolism and increasing your appetite. The purpose of these physiological adaptations is to slow the weight loss process and maintain the body's weight near its set point. This appears to be one logical explanation for the plateauing that follows initial weight loss.

While such factors as a steady high-fat/high-sugar diet are believed to raise the set point, it appears that your set point may be lowered, although the change can be expected to be long and slow. The two factors seeming to have the most significant effect in lowering set point are regular aerobic exercise (e.g., walking) and a diet high in complex carbohydrates (e.g., whole-grain breads and cereals, fruits, and vegetables).

Hormone (Insulin) Concept

Another factor that influences weight gain and weight loss is the activity of certain hormones in the body. Insulin, for example, is necessary for blood glucose (sugar) to be absorbed and utilized by body cells. When high-sugar foods are consumed, the body's immediate response is to release insulin into the bloodstream to regulate the body's blood sugar level. Following the

1. Calculate estimated unadjusted basal metabolic rate (BMR).

   a. Male: (Body Weight × 10) + (2 × Body Weight)

   b. Female: (Body Weight × 10) + Body Weight

2. To adjust the estimated BMR (from #1) for age, subtract 2% for each decade past 20's. For example, 2% if 30–39, 4% if 40–49, 6% if 50–59, 8% if 60–69, 10% if 70–79, etc.

3. To adjust the age-adjusted BMR (from #2) for body build, decide whether you are over or under standard weight, and estimate by how much (percentage). Then subtract (if overweight) or add (if underweight) the estimated percentage over or under.

   Example: If 10% overweight, subtract 10% from age-adjusted BMR.

   If 5% underweight, add 5% to age-adjusted BMR.

4. The answer in #3 is an estimated adjusted BMR (the number of calories needed to sustain life-supporting processes on a daily basis).

5. Calculate the estimated energy cost of daily light activity which includes digesting food, dressing, cooking, driving a car, and other basic daily activities.

   Adjusted BMR × 20% = Estimated energy cost for thermic effect of food and light activity

6. Calculate estimated pre-exercise metabolic rate (PXMR).

   Adjusted BMR (from #4) + 20% of BMR (from #5) = Estimated PXMR

7. Calculate estimated energy cost of all exercise activities. (See Table 10.1 for estimated energy cost of walking.)

8. Calculate estimated total metabolic rate (TMR), the total estimated energy cost (caloric expenditure) for all daily activities.

   Estimated TMR = RMR (from #6) + Exercise energy cost (from #7)

9. Estimated TMR is a calculated estimate of total energy (calorie) expenditure for a given day.

Figure 10.3 Estimating Daily Energy Expenditure

1. Calculate basal metabolic rate (BMR)

   a. Male: _____ + _____ = _____ cal.
            Body Wt. × 10   2 × Body Wt.   BMR

   a. Female: _____ + _____ = _____ cal.
            Body Wt. × 10   Body Wt.   BMR

2. Adjust BMR for age.

   _____ − _____ = _____ cal.
      Ans. #1   Age Adjustment   Age-Adjusted BMR

3. Adjust BMR for body build.

   _____ +/− _____ = _____ cal.
      Ans. #2   Wt. Adjustment   Adjusted BMR

4. Your adjusted basal metabolic rate is _____ cal./day
                           Ans. #3

5. Calculate energy cost for light daily activity.

   _____ × .20 = _____ cal.
      Ans. #4   TEF and Light Activity

6. Preexercising metabolic rate (PXMR)—Add 20% to adjusted BMR.

   _____ + _____ = _____ cal.
      Ans. #4   Ans. #5   PXMR

7. Calculate energy cost for all daily exercise (see Table 10.3).

   _____ _____ _____
    Exercise A   Exercise B   Exercise C

8. Total metabolic rate (TMR)—Add exercise energy expenditure to estimated PXMR.

   ____ + ____ + ____ + ____ = ____ cal.
  Ans. #6 Ans. #7a Ans. #7b Ans. #7c Est. TMR

9. Your estimated daily energy expenditure (TMR) is _____ cal./day
                           Ans. #8

Figure 10.4 Estimating Daily Energy Expenditure Worksheet

Table 10.1
Approximate Caloric Expenditure for Walking

Pace	Time	100	110	120	130	140	150	160	170	180	190	200	210	220	230	240	250
							Body Weight (lbs.)										
2.0 mph (30.00/mi)	30 min	57	63	69	75	81	86	90	96	102	108	114	120	126	131	137	143
	45 min	86	95	104	113	122	128	135	144	153	162	171	180	189	197	205	214
	60 min	114	126	138	150	162	171	180	192	204	216	228	240	252	262	274	285
2.5 mph (24.00/mi)	30 min	66	72	80	87	93	100	107	114	120	126	132	138	144	152	158	165
	45 min	99	108	119	131	140	150	161	171	180	189	198	207	216	228	238	248
	60 min	132	144	159	174	186	200	214	228	240	252	264	276	288	304	317	330
3.0 mph (20:00/mi)	30 min	75	84	90	98	105	113	120	128	135	143	150	158	165	173	180	188
	45 min	113	126	135	146	158	169	180	191	203	214	225	236	248	259	270	281
	60 min	150	168	180	195	210	225	240	255	270	285	300	315	330	345	360	375
3.5 mph (17:10/mi)	30 min	84	93	102	110	117	126	135	144	152	159	168	177	186	193	202	210
	45 min	126	140	153	164	176	189	203	216	227	239	252	266	279	290	302	315
	60 min	168	186	204	219	234	252	270	288	303	318	336	354	372	386	403	420
4.0 mph (15:00/mi)	30 min	111	123	134	144	156	168	179	189	201	212	222	234	246	255	266	278
	45 min	167	185	200	216	234	252	268	284	302	317	333	351	369	383	400	416
	60 min	222	246	267	288	312	336	357	378	402	423	444	468	492	510	533	555
4.5 mph (13:20/mi)	30 min	141	156	170	183	198	212	225	240	254	267	282	299	309	324	338	353
	45 min	212	234	254	275	297	317	338	360	380	401	423	448	464	486	508	529
	60 min	282	312	339	366	396	423	450	480	507	534	564	597	618	649	677	705
5.0 mph (12:00/mi)	30 min	180	198	216	234	252	270	288	306	324	342	360	378	396	414	432	450
	45 min	270	297	324	351	378	405	432	459	486	514	540	567	594	621	648	675
	60 min	360	396	432	468	504	540	576	612	648	684	720	756	792	828	864	900

digestion and absorption of sugar, blood insulin levels may remain elevated for some time. Increased blood insulin may increase hunger and possibly even the desire for sweets. If this is true, it can conceivably result in the desire for and consumption of additional carbohydrate and fat calories commonly found in sweet snack foods.

Such factors as eating high-sugar foods, being overfat (which requires the body to release even more insulin), eating a few large meals each day, and even seeing or smelling certain foods (candy, pastry, etc.) are thought to increase insulin activity, thus producing the increased desire for high-calorie foods. On the other hand, eating several smaller meals each day, enjoying a diet high in complex carbohydrates, and engaging in regular aerobic exercise will decrease insulin activity and, hopefully, help you control your sweet tooth.

Fat Cell Concept

Everyone has millions of specialized body cells (adipose) that are designed to store fat. Research indicates that obese people may have significantly more of these fat cells than nonobese people. Whether this is the result of genetics (an inherited trait) or environment (caused by diet, lack of exercise, etc.) is not

Table 10.2
Calculating Caloric Expenditure for Walking

The following table may be used to calculate the approximate caloric expenditure for walking at paces between 2.0 and 5.0 miles per hour:

Kcals Expended	=	Pace Factor (Kcal/lb/min)	×	Minutes walked	×	Body Weight (in pounds)

Pace (mph)	Pace Factor (Kcal/lb/min)	Pace (mph)	Pace Factor (Kcal/lb/min)
2.0	.019	3.6	.029
2.1	.019	3.7	.031
2.2	.020	3.8	.033
2.3	.020	3.9	.035
2.4	.021	4.0	.037
2.5	.022	4.1	.039
2.6	.023	4.2	.041
2.7	.023	4.3	.043
2.8	.024	4.4	.045
2.9	.024	4.5	.047
3.0	.025	4.6	.049
3.1	.025	4.7	.051
3.2	.026	4.8	.054
3.3	.026	4.9	0.57
3.4	.027	5.0	.060
3.5	.028		

Example: If you weigh 150 pounds and walk for 30 minutes at a pace of 3.5 miles per hour (pace factor of .028), you will burn approximately 126 Calories.

Kcals	=	Pace Factor	×	Minutes Walked	×	Body Weight
126	=	0.28	×	30	×	150

clear, although it is probably a combination of both.

Adipose cells appear to increase rapidly during three stages: the last 3 months of fetal development prior to birth, the first year after birth, and the adolescent "growth spurt" that most of us experienced. Whether adipose cell numbers increase during adulthood is not certain, although recent studies indicate that they may.

Once adipose cells are in place, they do not disappear with weight loss but merely shrink. Therefore, the more adipose cells you have, the more difficult it may be to keep weight off, since adipose tissue that shrinks during weight loss can just as easily fill with fat again if you don't practice weight management maintenance.

Effective Weight Loss

Weight gain/loss is a complex process that is probably influenced by not just one but all of the factors discussed in the previous section—

as well as others yet to be identified through scientific research. Therefore, it is unrealistic to expect a crash diet or some miracle weight loss product to take weight off and keep it off. What, then, is the best strategy for losing and maintaining a desirable body weight?

Not all weight loss is "effective" weight loss. *Effective weight loss* may be defined as weight loss that (1) is the result of fat reduction and (2) can be maintained on a long-term basis (for a lifetime).

There are basically three ways in which you can lose pounds. The most common source of quick weight loss is *dehydration,* or the loss of body water. While this will produce a lower reading when you step on the scales, it represents weight that will be quickly regained, and, most important, it is potentially dangerous. If you diet without exercising, you may lose lean body tissue (muscle) that also will be reflected on the scale as weight loss, but this loss is undesirable because muscle tissue is healthy and contributes to a variety of vital body functions. The third possible source of weight loss is excess fat. Of the three, only fat loss results in an effective, positive change in body composition. In fact, the use of exercise in an attempt to lose weight often produces a mysterious, and often frustrating, result if the scales are your only concern. Exercise (especially strength training) often causes an increase in muscle tissue along with the loss of body fat. Since muscle is denser than fat (i.e., it weighs more), it is quite possible to lose fat yet not lose (and possibly even gain) weight. Just remember, the first goal of any weight loss program should be to reduce the body's fat, thus achieving a healthier body composition.

The second aspect of effective weight loss (and the second goal of any weight loss program) is to maintain a healthy weight over a lifetime. For many people, losing weight is no problem; they have done it numerous times. Losing weight, then regaining it (often gaining more than you lost), not only is frustrating but ultimately very stressful on the body. Therefore, once weight is lost, maintenance is critical.

Weight management is often a difficult and frustrating process. However, effective weight loss can be achieved and maintained. The guidelines in the following sections are suggested for effective weight management.

Effective Weight Loss Must Be Done Gradually

Weight that is lost rapidly is often the result of dehydration and is seldom kept off. As a rule of thumb, the more gradually weight is lost, the more likely it is to be the result of a positive change in body composition (lost fat), and the easier it will be to keep it off. Safe and effective weight loss should take place at a rate of no more than ½ to 1 pound per week. While this number may sound painfully slow, just remember, unwanted weight gain occurs over months and years, so effective weight loss cannot be expected to be quick. Furthermore, the recommended rate will enable you to lose 15 to 25 pounds in about six months, and do it effectively.

Effective Weight Loss Must Involve a Change in Caloric Intake

To create a favorable energy balance, the first step is usually a reduction in the number of calories consumed. Contrary to popular belief, this can be a relatively painless process. Simply eliminating a candy bar or a couple of soft drinks from the daily diet can lower calorie intake by 300 or so calories per day. When combined with the 200 (or more) calories burned on your daily walk, you can easily create a favorable energy balance of 500 calories per day.

For some people, the kind of calories, in addition to the number, may need to be changed. Although the body can convert protein and carbohydrates into stored fat, it is dietary fat that contributes most directly to excess fat stores in the body. Since fats (9 calories/gram) are more than twice as calorie-rich as protein and carbohydrates (4 calories/gram each), eating equal amounts of protein, carbohydrates, and fats does not result in equal calorie intake. Simply stated, reducing dietary fat (even if some protein and/or carbohydrates are substituted in its place) may be the first step to a healthier diet. Also, as noted in the previous discussion of weight gain/loss concepts, increasing the amount of complex carbohydrates (starches) while reducing the amount of simple carbohydrates (sugars) may, without a significant reduction in carbohydrate calories, contribute to desired weight loss, since high-sugar foods are frequently also high in fat.

Effective Weight Loss Must Include Regular Exercise

As stated previously, dieting without exercise simply does not work. Not only may dieting without exercising lead to the unwanted loss of muscle tissue, but it also is very much like going into battle with one arm tied behind you. Regular exercise contributes to effective weight loss in a variety of ways. Strength training (lifting weights) increases not only muscle strength but also muscle size. Because muscle tissue is metabolically active (as opposed to fat), the result is a higher resting metabolism and, therefore, greater energy expenditure.

The best exercise for effective weight loss and maintenance, however, is aerobic exercise—and what better aerobic exercise than walking? Aerobic exercise is an effective way to burn calories, because it can be done comfortably for 30 to 60 minutes or longer. A 150-pound person will burn approximately 225 calories by walking 3 miles in 60 minutes. As your aerobic fitness improves, you will experience an increase in BMR, which means more calories burned at rest. Also, body fat is a major energy source during aerobic activity, and the more aerobically fit you become, the more efficiently your body will utilize (rather than store) fats. Contrary to popular belief, for some people, vigorous aerobic exercise such as fitness walking can actually result in a decreased appetite for 30 minutes or more following the exercise. Finally, as discussed earlier, regular aerobic exercise may help lower your set point as well as decrease insulin activity. So, for a variety of reasons, walking can be a key factor in effective weight loss and maintenance.

Effective Weight Loss Must Be Done Safely and Reasonably

The safest path to effective weight loss is a combination of sound nutrition and regular exercise. Fad diets that promise quick weight loss by eating only this food or none of that food are ineffective, a waste of time, and potentially dangerous. Even if a bizarre diet does result in weight loss, maintenance is virtually impossible because the diet cannot be tolerated for more than a few days. Likewise, weight lost by exercising in a heated environment or while wearing heat-trapping clothing is at best temporary and at worst potentially dangerous. There are no magic weight loss diets, pills, or potions.

When you purchase one of the "miracle weight loss products," the only significant weight loss will be to your pocketbook.

Effective Weight Loss Must Involve a Lifetime, Lifestyle Commitment to Maintenance

Weight loss that is not maintained is of little benefit. The key to long-term maintenance is your commitment to a healthy lifestyle that includes regular exercise and proper nutrition—and keeping that commitment for a lifetime.

Summary

It has been said that more Americans die of too much food than too little. Excess body fat is a major contributing factor in a host of health problems, not the least of which is cardiovascular disease. It appears that both our genetic makeup and the environment in which we live influence our tendency to gain weight. While energy balance (calories eaten versus energy expended) plays a major role in determining body composition, other factors such as personal set point, hormone balance, and adipose cell numbers also may be involved. You should strive to attain and maintain a desirable body composition through proper nutrition and regular exercise. If weight loss is your goal, remember that effective weight loss (fat loss) must (1) be done gradually; (2) involve a modification in caloric intake; (3) include regular exercise, such as walking; (4) be done safely and reasonably; and (5) result in a lifetime, lifestyle commitment to maintenance.

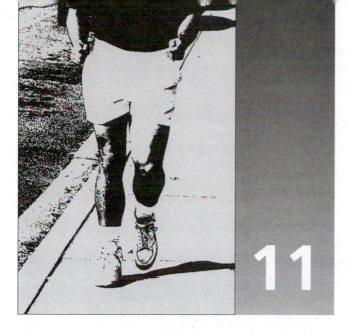

For you, as well as I, can open fence doors and walk across America in your own special way. Then we can all discover who our neighbors are.

Rob Sweetgall

11

Resources for the Fitness Walker

As you develop your own personal walking program, you will find that it is a process that is never really finished. An exciting and enjoyable walking program must be modified to meet your changing needs and interests. As you search for new ideas for maximizing the benefits of your walking program, you will find a wide variety of useful resources available. Among these are "canned" or predesigned walking programs, as well as numerous publications and Internet sites on walking, nutrition, weight management, and other wellness topics.

Walking Programs

Several well-known walking programs are available for those who prefer a preplanned program rather than developing their own. Many of these programs suggest a pretest to determine your beginning fitness level and then offer recommended programs based on your pretest results.

Rockport Walking Programs

The Rockport Company, a major manufacturer of walking shoes, has developed progressive walking programs for beginning, intermediate, and advanced walkers. Information on the Rockport walking programs may be obtained by contacting:

Rockport
220 Donald Lynch Blvd.
Marlboro, MA 01752
(800) 343-9255
www.rockport.com

Reebok Walking Programs

Reebok International Ltd., another major sports footwear manufacturer, also has fitness walking programs. The Reebok walking programs are based on the Personalized Aerobic Lifestyle System originally developed by the Aerobics Institute in Dallas, Texas. For information on Reebok walking programs, contact:

Reebok Offer
PO Box 4120
Huntington Station, NY 11746
(800) 843-4444

American Heart Association Walking Programs

The American Heart Association's Walking for a Healthy Heart program is designed primarily for beginning walkers. Information on this program may be obtained by contacting:

American Heart Association
    National Center
7320 Greenville Avenue
Dallas, TX 75231
(800) 242-8721
www.americanheart.org/catalog/
    health_catpage9.html

Walking and Fitness Publications

Walking Magazine
PO Box 5073
Harlan, IA 51593
(800) 829-5585
www.walkingmag.com

Dietary Guidelines for Americans
Superintendent of Documents
U.S. Government Printing Office
Washington, D.C. 20402
www.access.gpo.gov/su_docs

*University of California,
    Wellness Letter*
http://berkleywellness.com/

*Tufts University Health &
    Nutrition Letter*
www.healthletter.tufts.edu/

Walking Accessories

Cascade Designs, Inc. (hiking staffs)
4000 First Avenue South
Seattle, WA 98134
(800) 531-9531
www.cascadedesigns.com

Creative Health Products, Inc.
    (heart rate monitors)
1000 Saddle Ridge Road
Plymouth, MI 48170
(800) 742-4478
www.chponline.com

Exerstrider Products, Inc.
    (striding poles)
PO Box 3313
Madison, WI 53704
(800) 554-0989
www.exerstrider.com

Sports Music, Inc.
    (exercise tapes & CDs)
Dept. WM41A
Box 769689
Roswell, GA 30076
(800) 878-4764
www.sportsmusic.com

Web Sites of Interest

- Fitness walking information with a spiritual emphasis
  www.spiritedwalker.com
- Fitness walking information from coach Jake Jacobson
  www.healthwalk.com
- Fitness walking information from North Oaks Health System and Hammond Square Mall
  www.northoaks.org/ftf.html
- Fitness walking information
  http://trfn.clpgh.org/
- Fitness walking information from Meriter Health Services
  www.meriter.com/meriter/living/Library/sports/walknow.htm
- Health and fitness information from Covert Bailey
  www.healthcentral.com/fitorfat/fitorfat.cfm
- Information on fitness sites on the Internet
  www.fitnesslink.com/links.htm
- Wellness information from WELCUP Regional Fitness Council
  www.biz-commlcom/welcup
- Wellness information
  http://wellweb.com/

- Interactive wellness information from "Just Ask Alice" www.columbia.edu/cu/healthwise/
- Nutrition information http://nutrition.about.com/health/nutrition/msub3.htm
- Nutrition and fitness information from Ronda Gates www.rondagates.com/index2.html
- Information on nutrition myths http://206.74.57.36/zines/gourmet/articles/nutri.htm
- Information on nutrition sites on the Internet http://wce.uwyo.edu/wctl/high/nutr/default.html
- Weight control information www.CyberDiet.com/index.html
- Weight control information www.opendoor.com/IEHealth/FatLoss.html
- Weight control information www.shapeup.org/

Summary

Even though fitness walking is a relatively modern concept, numerous valuable resources are available to enhance the enjoyment of the beginning walker and experienced walker alike. A wide variety of pre-designed walking programs, books, periodicals, tapes, CDs, and Internet Web sites offer interesting information, as well as exciting ideas for keeping the fun in your walking.

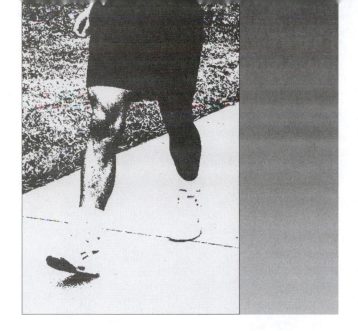

Appendices

Worksheets

Contents:

> These forms may be
> photocopied as necessary.

Appendix A

Calculating Target Heart Rate Range
Work Sheet

1. Determine predicted maximum heart rate (PMHR).

   a. Male: 210 – _____ = _____
                                 1/2 Your Age   PMHR

   b. Female: 220 – _____ = _____
                                   Age   PMHR

2. Take resting heart rate (RHR).   _____
                                               RHR

3. Subtract RHR from PMHR

   _____ – _____ = _____
             PMHR   RHR   Ans. #3

4. Multiply answer in #3 by 0.60 and 0.70:

   a. _____ x 0.60 = _____
              Ans. #3   Ans. #4a

   b. _____ x 0.70 = _____
              Ans. #3   Ans. #4b

5. To get target heart rate range (THRR), add answers in #4 to RHR:

   _____ + _____ = _____
             Ans. #4a   RHR   Lower THR

   _____ + _____ = _____
             Ans. #4b   RHR   Upper THR

Your target heart rate range (THRR) = _____ to _____

Appendix A

Calculating Target Heart Rate Range
Work Sheet

1. Determine predicted maximum heart rate (PMHR).

   a. Male: 210 − _____ = _____

    1/2 Your Age PMHR

   b. Female: 220 − _____ = _____

    Age PMHR

2. Take resting heart rate (RHR).   _____

    RHR

3. Subtract RHR from PMHR:

   _____ − _____ = _____

    PMHR $ $ RHR Ans. #3

4. Multiply answer in #3 by 0.60 and 0.70:

   a. _____ × 0.60 = _____

    Ans. #3 Ans. #4a

   b. _____ × 0.70 = _____

    Ans. #3 Ans. #4b

5. To get target heart rate range (THRR), add answers in #4 to RHR:

   _____ + _____ = _____

    Ans. #4a RHR Lower THR

   _____ + _____ = _____

    Ans. #4b RHR Upper THR

   Your target heart rate range (THRR) = _____ to _____

Appendix B

Personal Walking Accountability Plan

Name _____Date _____

Long-term Fitness Goal:

_____

_____

Short-term Performance Objectives:

1. _____

   _____

2. _____

   _____

3. _____

   _____

4. _____

   _____

Accountability Partner_____

Accountability Plan_____

_____

<table>
<tr><td>_____</td><td>_____</td></tr>
<tr><td align="center">Walker's Signature</td><td align="center">Partner's Signature</td></tr>
</table>

"Ideas are funny little things. They won't work unless you do."
Author Unknown

Appendix B

Personal Walking Accountability Plan

Name _____Date _____

Long-term Fitness Goal:

_____

_____

Short-term Performance Objectives:

1. _____

_____

2. _____

_____

3. _____

_____

4. _____

_____

Accountability Partner_____

Accountability Plan_____

_____

_____   _____
Walker's Signature   **Partner's Signature**

"Ideas are funny little things. They won't work unless you do."
Author Unknown

Appendix C

Estimating Your Daily Energy Expenditure

1. Calculate basal metabolic rate (BMR)

   a. Male: _____ + _____ = _____ cal.
   Body Wt. x 10   2 x Body Wt.   BMR

   b. Female: _____ + _____ = _____ cal.
   Body Wt. x 10   Body Wt.   BMR

2. Adjust BMR for age.

   _____ − _____ = _____ cal.
   Ans. #1   Age Adjustment   Age–Adjusted BMR

3. Adjust BMR for body build.

   _____ +/− _____ = _____ cal.
   Ans. #2   Wt. Adjustment   Adjusted BMR

4. Your adjusted basal metabolic rate is _____ cal./day
   Ans. #3

5. Calculate energy cost for light daily activity.

   _____ × .20 = _____ cal.
   Ans. #4   TEF and Light Activity

6. Preexercise metabolic rate (PXMR)—Add 20% to Adjusted BMR.

   _____ + _____ = _____ cal.
   Ans. #4   Ans. #5   PXMR

7. Calculate energy cost for all daily exercise (see Table 10.3).

   _____   _____   _____
   Exercise A   Exercise B   Exercise C

8. Total metabolic rate (TMR)—Add exercise energy expenditure to estimated PXMR.

   _____ + _____ + _____ + _____ = _____ cal.
   Ans. #6   Ans. #7a   Ans. #7b   Ans. #7c   Est. TMR

9. Your estimated daily energy expenditure (TMR) is _____ cal./day
   Ans. #8

Appendix C

Estimating Your Daily Energy Expenditure

1. Calculate basal metabolic rate (BMR)

   a. Male: _____ + _____ = _____ cal.
            Body Wt. x 10   2 x Body Wt.   BMR

   b. Female: _____ + _____ = _____ cal.
            Body Wt. x 10   Body Wt.   BMR

2. Adjust BMR for age.

   _____ − _____ = _____ cal.
       Ans. #1   Age Adjustment   Age–Adjusted BMR

3. Adjust BMR for body build.

   _____ +/− _____ = _____ cal.
       Ans. #2   Wt. Adjustment   Adjusted BMR

4. Your adjusted basal metabolic rate is _____ cal./day
                                     Ans. #3

5. Calculate energy cost for light daily activity.

   _____ × .20 = _____ cal.
       Ans. #4   TEF and Light Activity

6. Preexercise metabolic rate (PXMR)—Add 20% to Adjusted BMR.

   _____ + _____ = _____ cal.
       Ans. #4   Ans. #5   PXMR

7. Calculate energy cost for all daily exercise (see Table 10.3).

   _____   _____   _____
      Exercise A   Exercise B   Exercise C

8. Total metabolic rate (TMR)—Add exercise energy expenditure to estimated PXMR.

   _____ + _____ + _____ + _____ = _____ cal.
   Ans. #6   Ans. #7a   Ans. #7b   Ans. #7c   Est. TMR

9. Your estimated daily energy expenditure (TMR) is _____ cal./day
                                          Ans. #8

Appendix D

Walking Log

Name _____   **Week #1**

Date	Time	Distance	Pace	Calories	Comments
Total			XX		

Appendix D

Walking Log

Name _____   **Week #2**

Date	Time	Distance	Pace	Calories	Comments
Total			**XX**		

Appendix D

Walking Log

Name _____   **Week #3**

DATE	TIME	DISTANCE	PACE	CALORIES	COMMENTS
Total			**XX**		

Appendix D

Walking Log

Name _____　　　**Week #4**

Date	Time	Distance	Pace	Calories	Comments
Total			**XX**		

Appendix D

Walking Log

Name _____   **Week #5**

DATE	TIME	DISTANCE	PACE	CALORIES	COMMENTS
Total			XX		

Appendix D

Walking Log

Name _____   Week #6

Date	Time	Distance	Pace	Calories	Comments
Total			**XX**		

Appendix D

Walking Log

Name _____   **Week #7**

Date	Time	Distance	Pace	Calories	Comments
Total			**XX**		

Appendix D

Walking Log

Name _____   Week #8

Date	Time	Distance	Pace	Calories	Comments
Total			**XX**		

Appendix D

Walking Log

Name _____   **Week #9**

DATE	TIME	DISTANCE	PACE	CALORIES	COMMENTS
Total			**XX**		

Appendix D

Walking Log

Name _____   Week #10

Date	Time	Distance	Pace	Calories	Comments
Total			**XX**		

Appendix D

Walking Log

Name _____   **Week #11**

DATE	TIME	DISTANCE	PACE	CALORIES	COMMENTS
Total			**XX**		

Appendix D

Walking Log

Name _____   **Week #12**

Date	Time	Distance	Pace	Calories	Comments
Total			XX		